Exotic Animal Neurology

Editor

SUSAN E. OROSZ

VETERINARY CLINICS OF NORTH AMERICA: EXOTIC ANIMAL PRACTICE

www.vetexotic.theclinics.com

Consulting Editor
JÖRG MAYER

January 2018 • Volume 21 • Number 1

ELSEVIER

1600 John F. Kennedy Boulevard • Suite 1800 • Philadelphia, Pennsylvania, 19103-2899
http://www.vetexotic.theclinics.com

VETERINARY CLINICS OF NORTH AMERICA: EXOTIC ANIMAL PRACTICE Volume 21, Number 1
January 2018 ISSN 1094-9194, ISBN-13: 978-0-323-56661-2

Editor: Colleen Dietzler
Developmental Editor: Meredith Madeira

Veterinary Clinics of North America: Exotic Animal Practice (ISSN 1094-9194) is published in January, May, and September by Elsevier, Inc., 360 Park Avenue South, New York, NY 10010-1710. Subscription prices are $276.00 per year for US individuals, $492.00 per year for US institutions, $100.00 per year for US students and residents, $324.00 per year for Canadian individuals, $593.00 per year for Canadian institutions, $347.00 per year for international individuals, $593.00 per year for international institutions and $165.00 per year for Canadian and foreign students/residents. To receive student/resident rate, orders must be accompanied by name of affiliated institution, date of term, and the *signature* of program/residency coordinator on institution letterhead. Orders will be billed at individual rate until proof of status is received. Foreign air speed delivery is included in all *Clinics* subscription prices. All prices are subject to change without notice. **POSTMASTER:** Send address changes to *Veterinary Clinics of North America: Exotic Animal Practice*, Elsevier Health Sciences Division, Subscription Customer Service, 3251 Riverport Lane, Maryland Heights, MO 63043. **Customer Service: Telephone: 1-800-654-2452** (U.S. and Canada); **1-314-447-8871** (outside U.S. and Canada). **Fax: 1-314-447-8029. E-mail: journalscustomerservice-usa@elsevier.com (for print support); journalsonlinesupport-usa@elsevier.com (for online support).**

Reprints. For copies of 100 or more of articles in this publication, please contact the Commercial Reprints Department, Elsevier Inc., 360 Park Avenue South, New York, New York 10010-1710. Tel.: 212-633-3874; Fax: 212-633-3820; E-mail: reprints@elsevier.com.

Veterinary Clinics of North America: Exotic Animal Practice is covered in *MEDLINE/PubMed (Index Medicus).*

Contributors

CONSULTING EDITOR

JÖRG MAYER, Dr med vet, Msc
Diplomate, American Board of Veterinary Practitioners (Exotic Companion Mammals); Diplomate, European College of Zoological Medicine (Small Mammals); Diplomate, American College of Zoological Medicine; Associate Professor of Zoological Medicine, Department of Small Animal Medicine and Surgery, University of Georgia College of Veterinary Medicine, Athens, Georgia, USA

EDITOR

SUSAN E. OROSZ, PhD, DVM
Diplomate, American Board of Veterinary Practitioners (Avian); Diplomate, European College of Zoological Medicine (Avian); Bird & Exotic Pet Wellness Center, Toledo, Ohio, USA

AUTHORS

ROBERT D. DAHLHAUSEN, DVM, MS
Avian and Exotic Animal Medical Center, Veterinary Molecular Diagnostics, Inc, Milford, Ohio, USA

JAMIE M. DOUGLAS, DVM, MS
Postdoctoral Scholar, Department of Medicine and Epidemiology, UC Davis School of Veterinary Medicine, Davis, California, USA

PETER G. FISHER, DVM
Diplomate, American Board of Veterinary Practitioners (Exotic Companion Mammal Practice); Pet Care Veterinary Hospital, Virginia Beach, Virginia, USA

PAUL FLECKNELL, MA, VetMB, PhD, FRSB, FIAT (Hon), FRCVS (Hon)
Diplomate, European College of Laboratory Animal Medicine; Diplomate, Laboratory Animal Science; Diplomate, European College of Veterinary Anaesthesia and Analgesia; Diplomate, American College of Laboratory Animal Medicine (Hon); Emeritus Professor, Comparative Biology Centre, Medical School, Newcastle University, Newcastle, United Kingdom; Director, Flaire Consultants, Newcastle Upon Tyne, United Kingdom

LIVIO GALOSI, DVM
Animal Pathology Section, School of Biosciences and Veterinary Medicine, University of Camerino, Matelica, Italy

FRANK KÜNZEL, DVM, Dr, Priv Doz
Diplomate, European College of Zoological Medicine (Small Mammal); Clinical Department of Small Animals and Horses, University of Veterinary Medicine Vienna, Vienna, Austria

JAVIER G. NEVAREZ, DVM, PhD
Diplomate, American College of Zoological Medicine; Diplomate, European College of Zoological Medicine (Herpetology); Department of Veterinary Clinical Sciences, LSU School of Veterinary Medicine, Baton Rouge, Louisiana, USA

SUSAN E. OROSZ, PhD, DVM
Diplomate, American Board of Veterinary Practitioners (Avian); Diplomate, European College of Zoological Medicine (Avian); Bird & Exotic Pet Wellness Center, Toledo, Ohio, USA

MARY ANN OTTINGER, BS, MS, PhD
Department of Biology and Biochemistry, University of Houston, Houston, Texas, USA

JOANNE R. PAUL-MURPHY, DVM
Diplomate, American College of Zoological Medicine; Diplomate, American College of Animal Welfare; Professor, Department of Medicine and Epidemiology, UC Davis School of Veterinary Medicine, Davis, California, USA

SEAN M. PERRY, DVM
Department of Veterinary Clinical Sciences, LSU School of Veterinary Medicine, Baton Rouge, Louisiana, USA

GIACOMO ROSSI, DVM, PhD
Diplomate, European College of Zoological Medicine (Wildlife Population Health); Professor, Animal Pathology Section, School of Biosciences and Veterinary Medicine, University of Camerino, Matelica, Italy

DAVID SANCHEZ-MIGALLON GUZMAN, LV, MS
Diplomate, European College of Zoological Medicine (Avian, Small Mammal); Diplomate, American College of Zoological Medicine; Associate Professor of Clinical Zoological Companion Animal Medicine and Surgery, Department of Medicine and Epidemiology, UC Davis School of Veterinary Medicine, Davis, California, USA

JAN S. SUCHODOLSKI, MedVet, DrMedVet, PhD, AGAF
Diplomate, American College of Veterinary Microbiologists; Associate Professor, Small Animal Medicine, Associate Director for Research, Head of Microbiome Sciences, Gastrointestinal Laboratory, Department of Small Animal Clinical Sciences, Texas A&M University, College Station, Texas, USA

YVONNE VAN ZEELAND, DVM, MVR, PhD, CPBC
Diplomate, European College of Zoological Medicine (Avian, Small Mammal); Division of Zoological Medicine, Department of Clinical Sciences of Companion Animals, Faculty of Veterinary Medicine, Utrecht University, Utrecht, The Netherlands

LAURA L. WADE, DVM
Diplomate, American College of Veterinary Practitioners (Avian); Specialized Care for Avian & Exotic Pets, Clarence, New York, USA

Contents

> Reptiles have the anatomic and physiologic structures needed to detect and perceive pain. Reptiles are capable of demonstrating painful behaviors. Most of the available literature indicates pure μ-opioid receptor agonists are best to provide analgesia in reptiles. Multimodal analgesia should be practiced with every reptile patient when pain is anticipated. Further research is needed using different pain models to evaluate analgesic efficacy across reptile orders.

> This article reviews the current understanding of the anatomy and physiology of pain in birds, with consideration of some of its differences from mammalian pain. From transduction to transmission, modulation, projection, and perception, birds possess the neurologic components necessary to respond to painful stimuli and they likely perceive pain in a manner similar to mammals. This article also describes the current understating of opioid receptors, inflammatory mediators, and additional factors in the modulation of pain in avian species.

> Avian ganglioneuritis (AG) comprises one of the most intricate pathologies in avian medicine and is researched worldwide. Avian bornavirus (ABV) has been shown to be a causative agent of proventricular dilatation disease in birds. The avian Bornaviridae represent a genetically diverse group of viruses that are widely distributed in captive and wild populations around the world. ABV and other infective agents are implicated as a cause of the autoimmune pathology that leads to AG, similar to human Guillain Barrè syndrome. Management of affected birds is beneficial and currently centered at reducing neurologic inflammation, managing secondary complications, and providing nutritional support.

> Central vestibular dysfunction caused by *Encephalitozoon cuniculi* frequently mimics the condition of a peripheral disorder. A negative antibody titer rules out *E cuniculi* as the cause of present clinical signs. Cerebrospinal

fluid analysis, including polymerase chain reaction, is considered an inappropriate diagnostic method for in vivo diagnosis of encephalitozoonosis. The usefulness of glucocorticoid anti-inflammatories in the treatment of encephalitozoonosis is called into question. Encouraging activity early in the course of disease and adding in therapeutic exercise may represent the most important part of therapy in rabbits with vestibular dysfunction associated with encephalitozoonosis.

Managing pain effectively in any species is challenging, but small mammals present particular problems. Methods of pain assessment are still under development in these species, so the efficacy of analgesic therapy cannot be evaluated fully. Methods of assessing abdominal pain are established; however, applying these can be challenging. Alternative methods, using assessment of facial expression, may be more applicable to a range of painful procedures and across species. Multimodal and preventive analgesic strategies are most likely to be effective. Although data on analgesic dose rates are limited, sufficient information is available to enable analgesia to be provided safely.

Companion ferrets need to be vaccinated against 2 viral diseases that cause neurologic illness: canine distemper and rabies. Although not common in ferrets, both viruses are fatal in ferrets and rabies virus is also fatal in humans. In this article, we provide a basic review of the 2 diseases, highlighting key neurologic concerns. We also review and update current vaccine concerns from a practitioner's perspective, including available vaccines, vaccine schedule recommendations, vaccine reactions, and risk assessment. Last, we mention the ferret and its use in cutting-edge vaccine development.

The use of behavior-modifying drugs may be considered in birds with behavior problems, especially those refractory to behavior-modification therapy and environmental management. To accomplish behavior change, a variety of drugs can be used, including psychoactive drugs, hormones, antihistamines, analgesics, and anticonvulsants. Because their prescription to birds is off-label, these drugs are considered appropriate only when a sound rationale can be provided for their use. This requires a (correct) behavioral diagnosis to be established. In addition, regular monitoring and follow-up are warranted to determine the efficacy of the treatment and evaluate the occurrence of potential adverse side effects.

Avian species show variation in longevity, habitat, physiologic characteristics, and lifetime endocrine patterns. Lifetime reproductive and metabolic function vary. Much is known about the neurobiology of the song system in many altricial birds. Little is known about aging in neural systems in birds. Captive birds often survive beyond the age they would in the wild, providing an opportunity to gain an understanding of the physiologic and neural changes. This article reviews the available information with the goal of capturing areas of potential investigation into gaps in our under-standing of neural aging as reflected in physiologic, endocrine, and cogni-tive aging.

Jan S. Suchodolski

This article provides a brief overview of the advances made in microbiota research in parrots and pet birds. It describes this complex ecosystem and the contribution of the intestinal microbiota to host health and disease, including the nervous system.

VETERINARY CLINICS OF NORTH AMERICA: EXOTIC ANIMAL PRACTICE

ISSUE OF RELATED INTEREST

THE CLINICS ARE NOW AVAILABLE ONLINE!
Access your subscription at:
www.theclinics.com

Preface

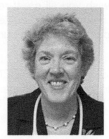

Susan E. Orosz, PhD, DVM, DABVP (Avian),
DECZM (Avian)
Editor

Neurology is an exciting area of study that is rapidly expanding its focus from humans to our exotic pets. As a student of neuroanatomy long ago, I was taught the classical view of vertebrate evolution of the brain. Based in part on Darwin's theory of evolution, it was theorized by Edinger and others that the evolution of the brain was linear and progressive, moving first from "lower" species that included fish to reptiles, then to birds, and then mammals. Humans were seen to represent the pinnacle of "brain-power!" This ascending order of intelligence could be traced back in part to the notion that the more intelligent brains retained some of these "primitive" parts, and the evolutionary view that increased intelligence came with an increase in complexity and size. This way of thinking influenced the naming of the structures of the brains of reptiles, birds, and mammals and hence the understanding of their intelligence. The traditional view suggested that reptiles and birds relied on those primitive components of the brain that were more instinctual and that, for these lower species, intelligent thought was not really possible: they just did not have the neuroanatomic structures to do that! In addition, the lack of a mammalian cortex suggested that reptiles and birds did not perceive pain. From a clinical perspective, this view hindered progression of our knowledge to enhance the lives of our exotic patients. The Brain Nomenclature Consortium has since looked deeply into the brains of the types of animals exotic animal veterinarians care for daily. They have provided a more modern view with a richer understanding of not only the organization of the brain but also the knowledge that these "lower species" have the ability to perceive pain and to think.

In the past, *Veterinary Clinics of North America: Exotic Animal Practice* has focused on understanding the components of neurologic exams in a variety of species. For this issue, I have given authors a voice on new and exciting and diverse topics that relate to the brain, from articles on pain in exotic animal species to the gut-brain barrier and understanding the aging brain of birds. Several of the authors have provided us with information on the neuroanatomic tracts that send pain information and where pain is perceived in the brain; these insights will certainly help us make our patients more comfortable.

Vet Clin Exot Anim 21 (2018) ix–x
https://doi.org/10.1016/j.cvex.2017.10.001
1094-9194/18/© 2017 Published by Elsevier Inc.

These articles provide timely information with clinical appeal for the readership on a variety of topics relating to the brain and to its health and disease. I appreciate the time and effort of each of the authors, who were willing to share their expertise in this exciting new frontier despite already full schedules. I wish you all great reading as you gain insights into the complexity of your patient's neurological faculties. As we learn more about the brain, we will continue to advance our ability to help our patients. Happy reading.

Susan E. Orosz, PhD, DVM, DABVP (Avian), DECZM (Avian)
Bird and Exotic Pet Wellness Center
5166 Monroe Street, Suite 306
Toledo, OH 43623, USA

E-mail address:
drsusanorosz@aol.com

Pain and Its Control in Reptiles

Sean M. Perry, DVM*, Javier G. Nevarez, DVM, PhD, DACZM, DECZM (Herpetology)

KEYWORDS

• Pain • Reptiles • Analgesia • Nociception • Multimodal analgesia • Opioid

KEY POINTS

• Reptiles have the anatomic and physiologic structures needed to detect and perceive pain.
• Reptiles are capable of demonstrating painful behaviors.
• Most of the available literature indicates pure μ-opioid receptor agonists are best to provide analgesia in reptiles.
• Multimodal analgesia should be practiced with every reptile patient when pain is anticipated.
• Further research is needed using different pain models to evaluate analgesic efficacy across reptile orders.

INTRODUCTION

Nociception is the processing of information by the peripheral and central nervous system (CNS) about internal or external stimuli to the body. Pain implies processing of this information at the level of the brain, specifically the cortex. In human terms, pain is the conscious perception of nociception as an unpleasant or adverse effect. Controversy has existed on whether nonmammalian species, such as reptiles, have the central and peripheral nervous system components to receive and process noxious stimuli as pain. Differentiating between a reptile "feeling" pain and having a "reflexive" response to noxious stimuli, or nociception, is at the crux of the pain debate in reptiles. Sound scientific data about the neuroanatomic, neurophysiologic, and behavioral pathways in reptiles are not as readily available as for other species and are often found in nonveterinary journals. Nonetheless, it has become a standard of practice to presume that reptiles are indeed capable of feeling pain and that analgesia should be an integral part of reptile medicine.

Disclosure Statement: The authors have nothing to disclose.
Department of Veterinary Clinical Sciences, Louisiana State University, School of Veterinary Medicine, Skip Bertman Drive, Baton Rouge, LA 70803, USA
* Corresponding author.
E-mail address: seanmperry87@gmail.com

NEUROANATOMY AND NEUROPHYSIOLOGY

The pathways required for pain processing include transduction, transmission, modulation, projection, and perception. All 5 categories are required components for the processing of pain by the brain.

Transduction

Transduction is the ability to detect innocuous to noxious stimuli within the environment by specialized or free nerve endings and transform them into action potentials. Like mammals, reptiles have cutaneous myelinated and unmyelinated afferent fibers running together in sensory nerves. Types of sensory nerves include myelinated A fibers (Aβ), small myelinated A fibers (Aδ), and small unmyelinated C fibers (C).[1,2] Additional documented peripheral receptors to aid in transduction have not been as well characterized compared with other vertebrates. Peripheral receptors may include intraepidermal mechanoreceptors, connective tissue mechanoreceptors without Schwann cell specializations, mechanoreceptors with Schwann cells, Merkel complexes, tactile sense organs, complex sensory organs, joint capsule endings, and sensory endings associated within the perichondrium, periosteum, tendons, and muscles. Reptiles, compared with other vertebrates, have relatively large terminal expansions of free nerve endings in the epithelial cells of the epidermis termed intraepidermal mechanoreceptors. Complex unencapsulated nerve endings occur in reptiles as in anamniotes, and they are characterized by an unmyelinated receptor axon in contact with surrounding connective tissue. A study in a pit viper species reported that Aβ fibers that respond to nonnoxious mechanical stimuli have a larger soma (cell body), whereas Aδ fibers that respond to noxious stimuli have a small soma, although there was no correlation with neuron function and soma size. Axon morphology was correlated with sensory neuronal function.[3] Substance P, a peptide neurotransmitter, documented within small afferent fibers, nerves, and dorsal and ventral horns of the spinal cord, is directly associated with painful stimuli in mammals. The substance P system is highly conserved across mammalian and nonmammalian species. In reptiles, substance P has been documented to occur within several turtle species.[4,5] Scant literature exists describing the required components to transduce painful or noxious stimuli in reptiles.

Transmission

Transmission occurs in the peripheral nervous system where action potentials occur and are transmitted to and from the spinal cord (CNS) and is then projected to the brain. Before being projected from the spinal cord to the brain, the signal in the form of action potentials can be modulated at the level of the spinal cord. Peripheral sensory nerve signals can be modulated, either amplified or suppressed, by interneurons present in the spinal cord. Specifically, the dorsal horn of the gray matter has interneurons that modulate the ascending neurons that receive, transmit, and project sensory information to the brain. Interneurons have been documented in the spinal cord of the red-eared slider (*Trachemys scripta elegans*) within the gray matter that assists in modulating movement and locomotion.[6,7] However, no studies have evaluated the role of interneurons and pain in reptiles.

Projection

Projection of sensory information from the periphery to the cerebral cortex within the spinal cord is a function of several ascending pathways originating from the spinal cord gray matter.[6,7] Axons of these pathways travel with the white matter of the spinal cord and terminate in higher centers within the brain, including the thalamus and reticular-activating system.[8] Three pathways exist in mammals that are responsible for transmitting painful and temperature-related sensations; these include the spino-thalamic, spinoreticular, and spinomesencephalic tract.[9] In reptiles, the same ascending pathways for auditory, visual, and somatosensory systems are present, but they have a reduced number of cell groups and subdivisions in the thalamus and pallium compared with mammals and birds.[10–15]

Perception

Perception is the integration, processing, and recognition of sensory information that occurs at multiple, different, specific areas of the brain that coordinate a response to painful or noxious stimuli. The reticular activating system in the brainstem is a critical center for the integration of sensory experiences and the subsequent affective and motivational aspects of pain through projections to the thalamus and limbic system. The periaqueductal gray matter (PAG) and thalamus serve as relay points for sensory information transfer, whereby the PAG relays sensory information to the thalamus and hypothalamus, whereas the thalamus transfers information to the cerebral cortex.

The telencephalon, which is the embryologic origin of the forebrain/cerebral cortex, consists of 2 subdivisions, the pallium and the basal ganglia. The basal ganglia are then further divided into the striatum and pallidum. These areas are thought to contribute to the septum and subpallial amygdala. The subpallial components are conserved in their distribution in amniotes.[15–17] The cerebral cortex in mammals is a derivative of the dorsal pallium. In mammals, the cerebral cortex is well developed. The dorsal pallium is homologous to the dorsal cortex in lizards and chelonians. All amniotes possess a dorsal pallium, which shares similar cell types and neuronal con-nections across different taxa.[15,18] The structure and organization of the reptile pallium has not been well established, although it is composed of the dorsal cortex, dorsal ventricular ridge, olfactory, hippocampal, and pallial amygdala regions. The anterior dorsal ventricular ridge in reptiles integrates information from many different sensory modalities and has a large number of projections into the striatum. In lizards, the ante-rior dorsal ventricular ridge is divided into 3 longitudinal zones, which process visual, somatosensory, and acoustic inputs. These inputs are relayed to the thalamic nuclei.[15,19]

In mammals, a characteristic of the forebrain is reciprocal connections between the thalamic nuclei and their cortical projections. In crocodilians, this feature is not present in the nuclei that project to the anterior dorsal ventricular ridge.[20,21] In crocodilians, telencephalic efferents arise from the basal ganglia. This pattern has been docu-mented in other reptiles and birds. However, in chelonians reciprocal connections be-tween the dorsal geniculate nucleus and the cortex have been documented.[20,22–24] The posterior dorsal ventricular ridge is considered the associative center that projects to the hypothalamus. This is comparable to the amygdaloid formation in mammals. The posterior dorsal ventricular ridge and surrounding structures compose the baso-lateral amygdala, the emotional portion of the brain. These structures have already been documented within ancestral amniotes. Based on this information, reptiles have the anatomic features necessary to feel or experience emotions based on anthropocentric views.[15,25]

In reptiles, descending motor pathways originating from the hypothalamus and brainstem to the spinal cord appear similar to mammals. Both chelonians (*Trachyemys scripta elegans* and *Testudo hermanni*) and lizards (*Varanus exanthematicus and Tupi-nambis nigropunctatus*) show similarities in their neuronal origin and spinal cord projection.[15,19] The interstitospinal, vestibulospinal, and reticulospinal tracts have been documented. In addition, the rubrospinal tract has been shown in some chelonians and squamates; however, it could not be demonstrated in a python species.[15] The absences of the rubrospinal tract is thought to be associated with limblessness, although it has been demonstrated in a water snake species *Nerodia* sp.[26] To determine if this is correlated with the loss of limbs, it might be beneficial to evaluate some lizard species thatho have undergone limb reduction.

The presence of a sensorimotor cortex in reptiles has only been documented in *Psammodromus algirus*, in which efferent fibers from the dorsal cortex reach the rostral midbrain tegmentum.[27] Similar corticoefferent pathways are described in chelonians after lesions in the cortex.[15,27] In Tokay geckos (*Geckko gecko*), anterograde-labeled fibers were present in the same tegmental region after tracers were injected into different locations in the dorsal cortex.[15,27] However, axon terminals were not observed in the Tokay gecko midbrain tegmentum. This strong evidence provides insight to the presence of a corticoreticulospinal motor pathway, which represents the anatomic pathway for the motor pallium in reptiles, which is comparable to the avian motor pallium, topologically and in regards to organization of efferent pathways.[27] In red-eared sliders, descending pathways linking cortical regions with the red nucleus via the hypothalamus is suggestive of indirect cortical control of the reptilian rubrospinal system.[27] Combining the information presented above suggests functionally segregated thalamocortical projections are conserved among amniote brain organization, thus providing evidence in reptiles that connections within the brain allow for pain perception pathways in the cortex to project to the thalamus. These cortical connections indicate the ability for reptiles to perceive pain, making it vital to provide adequate analgesia.

Based on the neuroanatomic comparisons between reptiles and other amniotes, there is enough information to presume that reptiles have the anatomic and physiologic capability to perceive pain. It must also be remembered than pain can be expressed differently across animal species; therefore, one should aim to err on the side of caution and always consider the use of analgesics in reptiles. Clinicians should use their best judgment and evaluate each case on an individual basis while also relying on current literature for up-to-date information. **Box 1** outlines some painful behaviors that reptiles have been known to exhibit. The remainder of this article empowers the clinicians to use evidence-based medicine to select the appropriate analgesics based on the latest information in the literature.

REPTILE ANALGESICS
Local Analgesics

Local anesthetics such as lidocaine and bupivacaine are used to inhibit peripheral nerve transmission and have the advantage of producing minimal systemic adverse effects at appropriate doses. Lidocaine, bupivacaine, and mepivacaine are often used in procedures that are considered minimally painful. Two studies have been published using local anesthetics in reptiles. A mandibular nerve block was performed using 2 anatomic approaches using a nerve locator and infusing mepivacaine perineuronally in 6 animals: 2 American alligators (*Alligator mississippiensis*), one dwarf crocodile (*Osteolaemus tetaspis*), and 3 yacare caiman (*Caman yacare*).[28] In Chinese box turtles (*Cuora flavomarginata*), lidocaine injection in the prefemoral region was insufficient as the sole anesthetic/analgesic method for performing endoscopic gender identification. Instead, the authors recommended general anesthesia to be used in conjunction with local anesthesia.[29]

Box 1
Painful behaviors in reptiles
Decreased to absent normal behaviors
Hunched posture
Decreased food intake
Lameness
Decreased activity
Decreased to absent interactive behaviors
Discoloration or skin-darkening of skin (chameleons and bearded dragons)
Rubbing affected area
Head carriage (extended or held away from the body)
Dull/closed eyes
Decreased tendency to coil (snakes)
Aerophagia
Aggressiveness in passive animals
Passive behavior in aggressive animals

Local anesthetics are thought to have conserved physiologic effect across species and vertebrate taxa because of their mechanism of action on neurons. However, reptile-specific information is not readily available, and no data exist on the evaluation of a toxic dose of local anesthetics in reptiles. Nonetheless, local anesthetics are commonly used in reptile patients with no apparent side effects reported.

Spinal Analgesia

Spinal analgesia usage in reptile practice is in its infancy. In mammals and humans, epidural anesthesia and spinal anesthesia are well established and commonly used for regional anesthesia of the spinal cord and nerves. Different classes of analgesics can be injected into the epidural or intrathecal space, which can result in inhibition of motor and sensory neurons as with local anesthetics, or sensory blockade with opioid analgesics. Spinal analgesia has only been described in the Galapagos tortoise and the red-eared slider.[30–32] A well-established clinical approach to the intrathecal space at the coccygeal vertebrae is described in **Box 2**. One report exists performing intrathecal injections at the atlanto-occipital joint in Marsh Terrapins (*Pelomedusa subrufa*).[33] The authors have no experience performing the latter approach; however, any analgesic that may inhibit motor function is not recommended at this level of the spinal cord to prevent paralysis.

Systemic Analgesics

Anti-inflammatories

Nonsteroidal anti-inflammatory drugs (NSAIDs) are the most widely used analgesics in reptilian practice, although few studies have evaluated the role of cyclooxygenase (COX) activity in the pathophysiology of pain and inflammation in reptiles.

In eastern box turtles (*Terrapene carolina carolina*), COX-1 and COX-2 expression was identified successfully in liver, kidney, and nontraumatized muscle tissue.[34]

Box 2
A step-by-step approach to intrathecal analgesia administration in chelonians

1. Mild sedation/anesthesia or manual restraint in a larger or cooperative patient.

2. Place animal in sternal recumbency and extrude the tail manually.

3. Aseptically prepare the dorsal tail.

4. Determine needle size based on animal size (Galapagos tortoise: 20-G needle, red-eared slider: 28-G needle).

5. Draw up local anesthetic or preservative free anesthetic drug.

6. Puncture skin and neural arch with the needle at a 45° angle.

7. Advance the needle into the spinal canal at a 20° angle.

8. Aspirate to ensure correct placement into the intrathecal space. Ensure an excessive amount of blood is not aspirated into the needle.

9. Administer drug over 3 to 5 seconds.

10. Evaluate limbs and tail for effects. Induction is seen within 5 minutes of injection. A repeat injection can be performed if there is no effect.

Note: Intrathecal catheters have been reported with this placement.

Adapted from Mans C. Clinical technique: intrathecal drug administration in turtles and tortoises. J Exot Pet Med 2014;23:67–70; and Rivera S, Divers SJ, Knafo SE, et al. Sterilisation of hybrid Galapagos tortoises (Geochelone nigra) for island restoration. Part 2: phallectomy of males under intrathecal anaesthesia with lidocaine. Vet Rec 2011;168:78.

Furthermore, this study compared COX-1 and COX-2 expression in traumatized muscle tissue to nontraumatized muscle tissue. COX-1 and COX-2 expression was increased in traumatized muscle tissue compared with nontraumatized muscle tissue. Although the COX-2 expression was noted to not be statistically significant, there was a 1.3- to 2-fold increase in COX-2 expression in traumatized tissue compared with nontraumatized tissue, which may still have clinical relevance. The highest levels of COX-1 and COX-2 expression were present in liver and kidney, although there was no statistically significant different between traumatized and nontraumatized tissues. This study successfully demonstrated COX expression in reptiles; however, it did not demonstrate the end products, such as PGE_2, TXA_2, $PGF_{2\alpha}$, PGD_2, or PGI_2, which are the primary mediators of inflammation and pain production associated with increased COX expression. Based on the expression pattern of COX-1 and COX-2 in traumatized and nontraumatized tissues in *T carolina*, the recommendation was to use nonselective rather than COX-2-selective NSAIDs.[34] In an experimental model using ball pythons, COX, NF-κB, ERK, and AKT signaling pathways were evaluated in inflamed and laser-induced inflamed skin and muscle.[35] Traumatized tissue was evaluated after induction of trauma using a CO_2 laser. This study showed COX-1 expression was increased in inflamed skin tissue compared with normal skin in the ball python, although there were no significant changes in the expression of either COX-1 or COX-2 in inflamed muscle tissue compared with normal muscle tissue. In addition, COX-2 production was not significantly greater in inflamed versus noninflamed skin and muscle specimens. They did observe evidence of inflammation and concurrent significant increases in production of other inflammatory signaling pathways, such as pERK in skin, and pERK and pAKT in muscle specimens.[35] These findings are similar to Royal and colleagues[34] suggestion of the use of nonselective COX inhibitors in ball pythons.

The current research on NSAIDs use in reptiles has evaluated the pharmacokinetics of meloxicam, a preferential COX-2 inhibitor. No pharmacodynamic studies are currently reported, and the data available do not provide strong evidence for their efficacy in reptiles. Oral administration of meloxicam to green iguanas (*Iguana iguana*) yielded excellent bioavailability, suggesting that plasma concentrations associated with analgesia in other species can be obtained for 24 hours after a single oral dose of 0.2 mg/kg.[36] In this study, no histopathologic changes were observed in renal, liver, or gastrointestinal tissue after 12 days of administration.[36] A dose of 0.2 mg/kg is also reported for intramuscular (IM) and intracoelomic administration in yellow-bellied sliders (*Trachemys scripta scripta*),[37] and IM and intravenous (IV) administration in red-eared sliders (*T scripta elegans*).[38] A dose of 0.1 mg/kg was reported to be inadequate for loggerhead sea turtles (*Caretta caretta*).[39] A dose of 0.3 mg/kg meloxicam did not provide analgesia in ball pythons (*Python regius*).[40]

Ketoprofen has been evaluated at 2 mg/kg IV in the green iguana and was determined to have a long half-life of 31 hours compared with ketoprofen in mammals. Based on these data, a dose of 2 mg/kg IV should be administered every 24 hours. However, the bioavailability after IM administration was only 78%, and its half-life is relatively short at 8.3 hours.[41] Ketoprofen has been used effectively in sea turtles at 2 mg/kg IM; however, duration of administration should be limited to 3 to 5 days.[42]

Further study of the reptilian inflammatory (**Fig. 1**) response is needed to identify the cellular response to injury and provide evidence-based information for therapeutic selection. Based on the current literature, the use of a nonselective COX inhibitor, such as Ketoprofen and Meloxicam, is preferred over selective ones. NSAIDs are not without deleterious side effects, although toxicities are not commonly reported from reptiles. They should be used with caution because of well-documented renal dysfunction, gastrointestinal ulceration, and thrombocytopathias reported in mammals and birds.

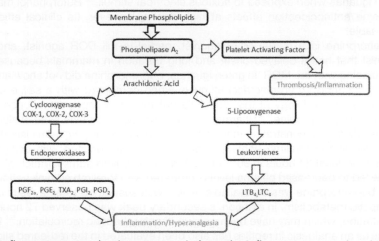

Fig. 1. Inflammatory cascade: tissue trauma induces the inflammatory cascade, which then releases prostaglandins and leukotrienes that can stimulate peripheral receptors at the tissue level to stimulate a painful sensation. Much of the primary scientific research determining the components in the inflammatory cascade has not been performed in reptiles. This is an extrapolation of what can be expected in the inflammatory cascade to be in reptiles.

Opioids

Opioids, the most commonly used analgesic in clinical practice, appear to be the most effective drug for controlling pain in reptiles. Opioids are classified based on their receptor subtypes, Mu (μ), Kappa (κ), and Delta (δ). A fourth subtype has been identified in mammals, nociceptin or orphanin FQ receptor; however, its implications in mammals are in question because studies investigating this receptor show mixed results.[43] The μ-receptors (MOR), κ-receptors (KOR), and δ-receptors (DOR), all mediate the analgesic effects of opioids. To further prove that opioids are effective analgesics in reptiles, identification of the receptor subtypes and their distribution within the CNS must be investigated. The opioid receptor gene family is highly conserved across several orders of vertebrates. Endogenous brain opiates have been identified in 2 snake species.[42] In red-eared sliders (*T scripta elegans*), both proencephalin-derived peptides and functional MOR, DOR have been identified in the brain.[43–46]

Evidence shows that MORs, KORs, and DORs are expressed in the reptile CNS. Butorphanol, a KOR agonist and a MOR antagonist, in other species is thought to only be a mild analgesic. The pattern has been observed in reptiles too, despite its frequent use. It is now accepted that butorphanol does not produce adequate antinociception in reptiles. Butorphanol in red-eared sliders (*T scripta elegans*) at a dose of 2.8 mg/kg and 28 mg/kg subcutaneously and in bearded dragons (*Pogona viticeps*) at a dose of 2 or 20 mg/kg did not show analgesic efficacy using a noxious thermal stimuli model. Butorphanol in corn snakes (*Elaphae gutatta*) showed a variable response, and the authors could not make any definitive conclusions.[47–49] Although the previously mentioned study evaluated butorphanol at 20 mg/kg, this dose was subsequently not recommended by one of the authors of the original publication in subsequent publications.[15] Other studies using butorphanol at 1 mg/kg IM in bearded dragons showed no analgesic efficacy, and there was no isoflurane-sparing effects in green iguanas (*I iguana*).[50,51] In ball pythons, butorphanol administered at 5 mg/kg IM had no analgesic effect on physiologic variables compared with a saline treatment group.[40] One study using butorphanol demonstrated that it may provide analgesia in green iguanas when exposed to noxious electrical stimuli.[52] Butorphanol may produce some antinociception effects at high doses; however, its clinical efficacy is questionable.

Buprenorphine is a partial MOR agonist, partial-to-full DOR agonist, and KOR antagonist that has a delayed onset and long duration in mammals because of its unique binding with the MOR. In green iguanas, buprenorphine did not show any antinociceptive effects to an electrical stimulus when compared with a saline control, although the methodology of this study did not take into account the longer onset of action of buprenorphine.[52] Pharmacokinetics of buprenorphine were evaluated in red-eared sliders demonstrating that a dose of 0.075 to 0.1 mg/kg administered subcutaneously in the forelimb achieves concentrations associated with analgesia in humans for at least 24 hours in 90% of the turtles. Hind limb administration of buprenorphine led to decreased plasma levels compared with forelimb administration. Only 70% of buprenorphine was bioavailable, which was suspected to be a result of first-pass hepatic metabolism. In addition, a secondary peak was observed 72 hours after administration, which may have been a result of enterohepatic recirculation.[53] Buprenorphine as an analgesic in reptiles has also been evaluated in the red-eared slider using a thermal noxious stimuli model at a dose of 0.1, 0.2, and 1 mg/kg subcutaneously. Buprenorphine failed to show a significant increase in hind limb withdrawal latencies at any time point when compared with saline between 3 hours and 96 hours after administration.[54] Based on current data, buprenorphine does not appear to be an efficacious analgesic in reptiles.

Pure MOR agonists have the most evidence supporting their use as analgesics in reptiles and are typically recommended as a first-line analgesic. Morphine sulfate was determined to be an effective analgesic in bearded dragons at 1 and 5 mg/kg and in red-eared sliders at 1.5 and 6.5 mg/kg using a thermal noxious stimuli model.[47–49] In corn snakes, morphine did not demonstrate efficacy even when administered at 40 mg/kg.[49] Morphine and meperidine provided analgesia in Speke's hingeback tortoises (Kinixys spekii) administered formalin into a limb and then reversed with naloxone after administration.[55] Morphine's analgesic efficacy in reptiles has been further supported by increased limb withdrawal latencies in crocodiles and increased tail flick latencies in anole lizards.[54–58] Another pure MOR agonist other than morphine that is commonly used in veterinary medicine is hydromorphone. This semisynthetic opioid is considered 5 times more potent than morphine. Hydromorphone administered at 0.5 mg/kg subcutaneously to the red-eared slider significantly increased hind limb withdrawal latencies using thermal noxious stimuli for up to 24 hours after administration.[52] Hydromorphone also appears to have less of a respiratory depression effect compared with morphine. Fentanyl is a pure MOR that is 75 to 100 times more potent than morphine. It can be administered to reptiles either transdermally or through an IV infusion. A study evaluating a fentanyl transdermally using a 12.5 μg/h patch in ball pythons (P regis) for 24 hours and corn snakes (E guttata) for 8 hours demonstrated the ability of fentanyl to be absorbed through reptilian skin.[59] In ball pythons, fentanyl reached plasma concentrations of 1 ng/mL within 4 hours of application of the fentanyl patch.[60] In the prehensile tailed skinks (Corucia zebrata), plasma fentanyl concentrations, using 10% exposure of total surface area of a 25 μg/h patch, were detectable by 4 to 6 hours and lasted for greater than 72 hours.[61]

Tramadol, a synthetic opioid analogue that acts as a μ-opioid agonist, has become a commonly used analgesic in veterinary medicine because it is readily available in an oral formulation. Its acceptance as an oral analgesic initially was due to the fact it was not listed as a controlled substance under the controlled substance act; however, as of 2014 tramadol has become listed as a schedule IV drug. Tramadol and its active metabolite O-desmethyltramadol produce analgesia by activating MOR and by inhibiting central serotonin and norepinephrine reuptake.[62,63] Tramadol in its parent form has MRO activity; however, the metabolite O-desmethyltramadol has up to 200 times greater affinity for MORs. Tramadol is converted into its more active metabolite O-desmethyltramadol in the liver. In mammals, there is controversy as to whether tramadol is an effective analgesic because some animals are unable to convert the parent form into O-desmethyltramadol in the liver, thus reducing its analgesic efficacy. In red-eared slider turtles, tramadol at 5 mg/kg orally significantly increased withdrawal latencies for 12 to 24 hours. At 10 mg/kg and 25 mg/kg, increased withdrawal latencies were observed up to 6 and 96 hours, respectively.[64] Pharmacokinetics of tramadol and its metabolite, O-desmethyltramadol, were evaluated following oral administration of 2 doses (5 mg/kg and 10 mg/kg) in the loggerhead sea turtle (Carretta carretta).[65] Tramadol and O-desmethyltramadol plasma concentrations remained greater than 100 ng/mL for at least 48 and 72 hours when administered at 10 mg/kg orally.[65] IM administration of tramadol at 10 mg/kg in the yellow-bellied slider (T scripta scripta) was evaluated in a placebo controlled crossover study evaluating injection site location.[66] They evaluated thermal withdrawal latency to evaluate the drug's effectiveness as an analgesic. The 2 pharmacokinetic profiles for tramadol differed in the first 2 hours following administration, but overlapped in the elimination phase. Tramadol's metabolite, O-desmethyltramadol, was formed in both hind limb and forelimb administration groups and showed a similar pharmacokinetic trend, although the metabolite was significantly higher, about 20%, in the hind limb group. The turtles in both forelimb and hind limb group showed a significant increase in thermal withdrawal latency over the periods of 0.5 to 48 hours and 8 to 48 hours, respectively. Plasma tramadol concentration and effect versus time curves were shown to not correlate. Although the O-desmethyltramadol concentration and effect time curves appear to not have a direct correlation, when antinociception effect was plotted against plasma O-desmethyltramadol, the plasma concentration and effect showed a counterclockwise hysteresis loop shape. This study demonstrated that tramadol injection into the hind limb may lead to faster therapeutic plasma concentrations of O-desmethyltramadol because of first pass hepatic metabolism.[66] Because O-desmethyltramadol is present in reptiles, it would suggest that it has potential for being an efficacious alternative. However, further studies are needed to fully assess tramadol efficacy in reptiles.

Tapentadol, a centrally acting MOR agonist and norepinephrine reuptake inhibitor, has been evaluated in yellow belly sliders (*T scripta scripta*) after a single IM injection at 5 mg/kg. In this study, the pharmacokinetics and pharmacodynamics of tapentadol were determined using high-performance liquid chromatography and thermal withdrawal latency times over a 24-hour period. Individuals receiving tapentadol showed an increase in thermal withdrawal latency starting at 1 hour after administration of tapentadol, and a linear relationship was observed between plasma concentrations and percent maximum possible response. Tapentadol was demonstrated to be efficacious in the yellow belly slider at 5 mg/kg IM.[67,68]

Many of the studies mentioned above use a single thermal model to evaluate antinociception in reptiles. This model appears to be reproducible and has become the standard. Validation of other models would provide additional support for the efficacy of these opioids in reptiles.

Other analgesics

Other well-established analgesics in human and veterinary medicine have hardly been used and explored in their application to herpetologic medicine, despite evidence that the functional anatomy and physiology are present within the reptilian brain.

α_2-ADRENERGIC AGONISTS

α_2-adrenergic agonists, in reptiles, are commonly used in conjunction with other analgesic medications primarily for the sedative effects. This class of anesthetics has been thought to have analgesic effects in reptiles because of the widely documented analgesic effects observed in humans and mammals. Only one study exists evaluating the analgesic properties of α_2-adrenergic agonists as an analgesic (**Table 1**). This study evaluated marsh terrapins' (*P subrufa*) pain-related behaviors following subcutaneous administration of 8% formalin. Animals were divided into control and treatment groups and administered intrathecal injections of clonidine (18.75 µg/kg, 37 µg/kg, and 65 µg/kg), yohimbine (25 µg/kg, 40 µg/kg, and 53 µg/kg), a combination of clonidine and yohimbine (65 µg/kg and 25 µg/kg), and methysergide maleate (20 µg/kg) and yohimbine (53 µg/kg). Clonidine used alone exhibited a dose-dependent decrease in pain-related behaviors when administered intrathecally. In addition, duration of pain-related behaviors was observed to decrease in animals treated with clonidine (65 µg/kg) exclusively when compared with groups of animals with yohimbine exclusively and yohimbine and clonidine. Animals that were given methysergide maleate and yohimbine demonstrated that treatment with yohimbine alone at (53 µg/kg) decreased pain-related behaviors. The use of methysergide maleate and yohimbine in this study suggests that the 5-HT neurotransmitter system may play a role in pain in chelonians; however, the study lacked a treatment group with methysergide

Table 1
Peer-reviewed analgesic medications

Medication	Dose (mg/kg)	Route	Species
Opioids			
Buprenorphine	0.075–0.1 0.02–0.1	IM, SC	Green iguana,[52] red-eared slider[53,54]
Butorphanol	0.4–8.0 1.0–20.0	IM, SC	Red-eared slider,[48,69] bearded dragon,[49] corn snake,[49] green iguana,[50–52] ball python[59]
Hydromorphone	0.5–1	IM, SC	Red-eared slider[54]
Fentanyl	12.5 µg/h 2.5 µg/h	Transdermal	Ball python,[60] corn snake,[59] prehensile tail skink[61]
Meperidine	1.0–5.0 10.0–50.0	IM, SC	Speke's hinge back tortoise,[55] red-eared slider, crocodilians[56]
Methadone	3.0–5.0	IM, SC	Green iguana[36]
Morphine	1.0–40.0	IM, SC, IT	Red-eared sliders,[48,69] bearded dragons,[49] crocodilians,[56] green iguana[52]
Tapentadol	5.0	IM	Yellow-belly slider[67]
Tramadol	5.0–10.0	PO	Loggerhead sea turtles,[65] red-eared sliders,[64] yellow-bellied slider[66]
NSAIDs			
Carprofen	1.0–4.0	SC, IM	Anecdotal[14]
Ketoprofen	2.0	IV	Green iguanas[41]
Meloxicam	0.2–0.3	IV, SC, IM, PO	Green iguanas,[36] ball pythons[40]
Local anesthetics			
Lidocaine	1–2 (keep <4) 4	SC, IM IT	Galapagos tortoise,[30] red-eared slider,[31,32] Chinese box turtles[29]
Bupivicaine	1.0 (keep <2) 1.0	SC, IM IT	Red-eared slider[31,32]
Mepivacaine	1.0	SC	Alligators[28]
Other possible analgesics			
Dexmeditomidine	0.1–0.2	SC, IM	Not yet evaluated for analgesic efficacy in reptiles, all doses extrapolated from mammalian literature[14]
Ketamine	2	SC, IM, IV	
Medetomidine	0.05–0.3	SC, IM	

Abbreviations: IT, intrathecal; PO, orally; SC, subcutaneous.

maleate, yohimbine, and clonidine, which would allow for stronger evidence for 5-HT neurotransmitter involvement.[33]

NMDA RECEPTOR ANTAGONIST

Low-dose usage of ketamine in other species, especially mammals, has been demonstrated to decrease analgesic requirements especially in the postoperative period. NMDA receptors play a central role in central sensitization and wind up providing analgesic properties. In addition, when used in concert with other medications such as opioids, ketamine can lower the dose requirements of other drugs (**Table 2**). In reptiles, no data are available to demonstrate ketamine's effectiveness as an analgesic. Increased sedation does occur when ketamine is used in conjunction with other

Table 2		
Commonly used medications and which opioid receptor subtypes they effect		
	Opioid Agonists	**Opioid Antagonists**
Mu (μ) receptor	Morphine, hydromorphone, fentanyl, methadone, oxymorphone, tramadol, tapentadol	Naloxone, naltrexone
Kappa (κ) receptor	Butorphanol (κ agonists/partial μ antagonists), nalbuphine (κ agonists/partial μ antagonists)	Naloxone, naltrexone
Delta (δ) receptor	All drugs are experimental at this time	Naltridole, naloxone, naltrexone

sedatives/analgesics. The analgesic effects of ketamine in reptiles can only be extrapolated until studies are performed.

Other analgesic drugs, such as gabapentin, amantadine, pregablin, mexiletine, alendronate, tricyclic antidepressants, nutraceuticals, and physical therapy/rehabilitation, have yet to be evaluated in reptiles, although many of these therapies could lead to a better understanding of nociception, pain, and analgesic therapy. Research is desperately needed so clinicians can make evidence-based therapeutic decisions when analgesia is required.

ALTERNATIVE MEDICINE

Acupuncture has been used as an analgesic in humans, dogs, horses, and rodents, but minimal data exist from controlled studies. In rats, electroacupuncture-induced analgesia is attributed to stimulation of MORs, KORs, and DORs. One study has transposed acupuncture points to a red-footed tortoise (*Chelonoidis carbonaria*) to treat a locomotor disability.[70] Electroacupuncture has been thought to act on MORs, which sets the possibility of its use as an adjunct analgesics modality. Bearded dragons treated with electroacupuncture may show a trend toward delayed limb withdrawal after exposure to thermal noxious stimuli, although the data are not considered to be statistically significant from the controls.[14]

PREEMPTIVE AND MULTIMODAL ANALGESIA

Analgesia in reptile patients is best achieved when inhibiting several different physiologic pathways that induce pain in addition to preemptively treating pain when a painful stimuli is anticipated. Multimodal analgesia indicates using multiple drugs in combination to attenuate or eliminate the physiologic signals from the peripheral nervous system to the CNS. Analgesics such as opioids act within the central and peripheral nervous system to alter the physiologic response of pain, whereas NSAIDs act at the tissue level rather than within the nervous system. Application of local anesthetics can inhibit initial transmission of pain in the peripheral nervous system. The synergistic effects of multimodal analgesia can only benefit the patients. Although no studies exist in reptiles evaluating the synergistic effects of multimodal analgesia, the authors advocate using multimodal analgesia whenever possible based on personal experience and extrapolation from other veterinary and human literature.

SUMMARY

Compared with the mammalian veterinary literature, the amount of information on reptile analgesia is very limited. Nonetheless, within the past 10 years, the reptile analgesia literature has expanded significantly. Reptiles possess the anatomic and physiologic structures needed to detect and perceive pain. In addition, they are capable of demonstrating painful behaviors like other species, such as mammals. Most of the available literature indicates pure μ-opioid receptor agonists are best to provide analgesia in reptiles, while nonselective COX inhibitors may be best to prevent inflammation to assist in controlling pain. Multimodal analgesia should be practiced in every reptile patient when pain or noxious stimuli is anticipated. Additional research is needed using different pain models to evaluate analgesic efficacy in the different reptile orders.

REFERENCES

1. Sneddon LU. Evolution of nociception in vertebrates: comparative analysis of lower vertebrates. Brain Res Rev 2004;46:123–30.
2. Stevens CW. Analgesia in amphibians: preclinical studies and clinical applications. Vet Clin North Am Exot Anim Pract 2011;14:33–44.
3. Liang YF, Terashima S, Zhu AQ. Distinct morphological characteristics of touch, temperature, and mechanical nociceptive neurons in the crotaline trigeminal ganglia. J Comp Neurol 1995;60:621–33.
4. Partata WA, Krepsky AMR, Xavier LL, et al. Substance P immunoreactivity in the lumbar spinal cord of the turtle Trachemys dorbigni following peripheral nerve injury. Braz J Med Biol Res 2003;36:515–20.
5. Reiner A, Krause JE, Keyser KT, et al. The distribution of substance P in turtle nervous system: a radioimmunoassay and immunohistochemical study. J Comp Neurol 1984;226:50–75.
6. Berkowitz A. Multifunctional and specialized spinal interneurons for turtle limb movements: multifunctional and specialized spinal interneurons. Ann N Y Acad Sci 2010;1198:119–32.
7. Berkowitz A. Physiology and morphology of shared and specialized spinal interneurons for locomotion and scratching. J Neurophysiol 2008;99:2887–901.
8. Mehler WR. Subcortical afferent connections of the amygdala in the monkey. J Comp Neurol 1980;190:733–62.
9. Willis WD. Nociceptive pathways: anatomy and physiology of nociceptive ascending pathways. Philos Trans R Soc Lond B Biol Sci 1985;308:253–70.
10. Hall WC, Ebner FF. Thalamotelencephalic projections in the turtle (Pseudemys scripta). J Comp Neurol 1970;140:101–22.
11. Bruce LL, Butler AB. Telencephalic connections in lizards. II. Projections to anterior dorsal ventricular ridge. J Comp Neurol 1984a;229:602–15.
12. Kenigfest N, Martínez-Marcos A, Belekhova M, et al. A lacertilian dorsal retinorecipient thalamus: a re-investigation in the old-world lizard Podarcis hispanica. Brain Behav Evol 1997;50:313–34.
13. Butler AB, Manger PR, Lindahl BI, et al. Evolution of the neural basis of consciousness: a bird-mammal comparison. Bioessays 2005;27:923–36.
14. Sladky KK. Analgesia. In: Mader DM, Divers SJ, editors. Current therapy in reptile medicine and surgery. St Louis (MO): Elsevier Inc; 2014. p. 217–28.
15. Butler AB, Hodos W. Comparative vertebrate neuroanatomy: evolution and adaptation. 2nd edition. Hoboken (NJ): John Wiley & Sons; 2005.
16. Jarvis ED. Evolution of the pallium in birds and reptiles. In: Binder MD, Hirokawa N, Windhorst U, editors. New encyclopedia of neuroscience. Berlin: Springer-Verlag GmbH; 2009. p. 1390–400.

17. Medina L, Abellán A. Development and evolution of the pallium. Semin Cell Dev Biol 2009;20:698–711.
18. ten Donkelaar HJ, de Boer-van Huizen R. A possible pain control system in a non-mammalian vertebrate (a lizard, Gekko gecko). Neurosci Lett 1987;83:65–70.
19. Pritz MB. Dorsal thalamic nuclei in Caiman crocodilus. Neurosci Lett 2014;58: 57–62.
20. Pritz MB. Crocodilian forebrain: evolution and development. Integr Comp Biol 2015;55:949–61.
21. Hall JA, Foster RE, Ebner FF, et al. Visual cortex in a reptile, the turtle (Pseudemys scripta and Chrysemys picta). Brain Res 1977;130:197–216.
22. Ulinski PS. Organization of corticogeniculate projections in the turtle, Pseudemys scripta. J Comp Neurol 1986;254:529–42.
23. Kenigfest NB, Repérant J, Rio JP, et al. Retinal and cortical afferents to the dorsal lateral geniculate nucleus of the turtle, Emys orbicularis: a combined axonal tracing, glutamate, and GABA immunocytochemical electron microscopic study. J Comp Neurol 1998;391:470–90.
24. Novejarque A, Lanuza E, Martínez-García F. Amygdalostriatal projections in reptiles: a tract-tracing study in the lizard Podarcis hispanica. J Comp Neurol 2004; 479:287–308.
25. Cruce WLR, Larson-Prior L, Newman DB. Rubrospinal pathways in a colubrid snake. Soc Neurosci Abstr 1983;9:1064.
26. Guirado S, Dávila JC. Thalamo-telencephalic connections: new insights on the cortical organization in reptiles. Brain Res Bull 2002;57:451–4.
27. Zhu D, Lustig KH, Bifulco K, et al. Thalamocortical connections in the pond turtle Pseudemys scripta elegans. Brain Behav Evol 2005;65:278–92.
28. Wellehan JFX, Gunkel CI, Kledzik D, et al. Use of a nerve locator to facilitate administration of mandibular nerve blocks in crocodilians. J Zoo Wildl Med 2006;37:405–8.
29. Hernandez-Divers SJ, Stahl SJ, Farrell R. An endoscopic method for identifying sex of hatchling Chinese box turtles and comparison of general versus local anesthesia for coelioscopy. J Am Vet Med Assoc 2009;234:800–4.
30. Rivera S, Divers SJ, Knafo SE, et al. Sterilisation of hybrid Galapagos tortoises (Geochelone nigra) for island restoration. Part 2: phallectomy of males under intrathecal anaesthesia with lidocaine. Vet Rec 2011;168:78.
31. Mans C, Steagall PVM, Lahner LL, et al. Efficacy of intrathecal lidocaine, bupivacaine, and morphine for spinal anesthesia and analgesia in red-eared slider turtles (Trachemys scripta elegans). Proc Am Assoc Zoo Vet 2011;135.
32. Mans C. Clinical technique: intrathecal drug administration in turtles and tortoises. J Exot Pet Med 2014;23:67–70.
33. Makau CM, Towett PK, Abelson KSP, et al. Intrathecal administration of clonidine or yohimbine decreases the nociceptive behavior caused by formalin injection in the marsh terrapin (Pelomedusa subrufa). Brain Behav 2014;4:850–7.
34. Royal LW, Lascelles BDX, Lewbart GA, et al. Evaluation of cyclooxygenase protein expression in traumatized versus normal tissues from eastern box turtles (Terrapene carolina carolina). J Zoo Wildl Med 2012;43:289–95.
35. Sadler RA, Schumacher JP, Rathore K, et al. Evaluation of the role of the cyclooxygenase signaling pathway during inflammation in skin and muscle tissues of ball pythons (Python regius). Am J Vet Res 2016;77:487–94.
36. Divers SJ, Papich M, McBride M, et al. Pharmacokinetics of meloxicam following intravenous and oral administration in green iguanas (Iguana iguana). Am J Vet Res 2010;71:1277–83.

37. Di Salvo A, Giorgi M, Catanzaro A, et al. Pharmacokinetic profiles of meloxicam in turtles (Trachemys scripta scripta) after single oral, intracoelomic and intramuscular administrations. J Vet Pharmacol Ther 2016;39(1):102–5.
38. Uney K, Altan F, Aboubakr M, et al. Pharmacokinetics of meloxicam in red-eared slider turtles (Trachemys scripta elegans) after single intravenous and intramuscular injections. Am J Vet Res 2016;77(5):439–44.
39. Lai OR, Di Bello A, Soloperto S, et al. Pharmacokinetic behavior of meloxicam in loggerhead sea turtles (Caretta caretta) after intramuscular and intravenous administration. J Wildl Dis 2015;51(2):509–12.
40. Olesen MG, Bertelsen MF, Perry SF, et al. Effects of preoperative administration of butorphanol or meloxicam on physiologic responses to surgery in ball pythons. J Am Vet Med Assoc 2008;233:1883–8.
41. Tuttle AD, Papich M, Lewbart GA, et al. Pharmacokinetics of ketoprofen in the green iguana (Iguana iguana) following single intravenous and intramuscular injections. J Zoo Wildl Med 2006;37:567–70.
42. Hannon D. Non-steroidal anti-inflammatory drugs (NSAIDs) in reptiles and amphibians: a review. Proc Exoticscon 2015;589–603.
43. Stevens CW. The evolution of vertebrate opioid receptors. Front Biosci 2009;14:1247–69.
44. Ng TB, Ng ASL, Wong CC. Adrenocorticotropin-like and beta-endorphin-like substances in brains of the fresh-water snake Ptyas mucosa. Biochem Cell Biol 1990;68:1012–8.
45. Xia Y, Haddad GG. Major difference in the expression of delta- and mu-opioid receptors between turtle and rat brain. J Comp Neurol 2001;436:202–10.
46. Reiner A. The distribution of proenkephalin-derived peptides in the central nervous system of turtles. J Comp Neurol 1987;259:65–91.
47. Sladky KK, Kinney ME, Johnson SM. Effects of opioid receptor activation on thermal antinociception in red-eared slider turtles (Trachemys scripta). Am J Vet Res 2009;70:1072–8.
48. Sladky KK, Miletic V, Paul-Murphy J, et al. Analgesic efficacy and respiratory effects of butorphanol and morphine in turtles. J Am Vet Med Assoc 2007;230:1356–62.
49. Sladky KK, Kinney ME, Johnson SM. Analgesic efficacy of butorphanol and morphine in bearded dragons and corn snakes. J Am Vet Med Assoc 2008;233:267–73.
50. Fleming GJ, Robertson SA. Assessments of thermal antinociceptive effects of butorphanol and human observer effect on quantitative evaluation of analgesia in green iguanas (Iguana iguana). Am J Vet Res 2012;73:1507–11.
51. Mosley CA, Dyson D, Smith DA. Minimum alveolar concentration of isoflurane in green iguanas and the effect of butorphanol on minimum alveolar concentration. J Am Vet Med Assoc 2003;222:1559–64.
52. Greenacre CB, Schumacher JP, Talke G, et al. Comparative antinociception of morphine, butorphanol, and buprenorphine versus saline in the green iguana, Iguana iguana, using electrostimulation. J Herpetol Med Surg 2006;16:88–92.
53. Kummrow MS, Tseng F, Hesse L, et al. Pharmacokinetics of buprenorphine after single-dose subcutaneous administration in red-eared sliders (Trachemys scripta elegans). J Zoo Wildl Med 2008;39:590–5.
54. Mans C, Lahner LL, Baker BB, et al. Antinociceptive efficacy of buprenorphine and hydromorphone in red-eared slider turtles (Trachemys scripta elegans). J Zoo Wildl Med 2012;43:662–5.

55. Wambugu SN, Towett PK, Kiama SG, et al. Effects of opioids in the formalin test in the Speke's hinged tortoise (Kinixys spekii). J Vet Pharmacol Ther 2010;33: 347–51.

56. Kanui TI, Hole K. Morphine and pethidine antinociception in the crocodile. J Vet Pharmacol Ther 1992;15:101–3.

57. Kanui TI, Hole K, Miaron JO. Nociception in crocodiles—capsaicin instillation, formalin and hot plate tests. Zool Sci 1990;7:537–40.

58. Mauk MD, Olson RD, Lahoste GJ, et al. Tonic immobility produces hyperalgesia and antagonizes morphine analgesia. Science 1981;213:353–4.

59. Gutwillig A, Abbott A, Johnson SM, et al. Opioid dependent analgesia in ball pythons (Python regius) and corn snakes (Elaphe guttata). Proc Assoc Reptile Amphibian Vets 2012;66.

60. Darrow BG, Meyers GE, Kukanich B. Fentanyl transdermal therapeutic system pharmacokinetics in ball pythons (Python regius). Proc Am Assoc Zoo Vet 2010;238–9.

61. Gamble KC. Plasma fentanyl concentrations achieved after transdermal fentanyl patch application in prehensile-tailed skinks, Corucia zebrata. J Herpetol Med Surg 2008;18:81–5.

62. Raffa RB, Friderichs E, Reimann W, et al. Opioid and nonopioid components independently contribute to the mechanism of action of tramadol, an atypical opioid analgesic. J Pharmacol Exp Ther 1992;260:275–85.

63. Ide S, Minami M, Ishihara K, et al. Mu opioid receptor-dependent and independent components in effects of tramadol. Neuropharmacology 2006;51:651–8.

64. Baker BB, Sladky KK, Johnson SM. Evaluation of the analgesic effects of oral and subcutaneous tramadol administration in red-eared slider turtles. J Am Vet Med Assoc 2011;238:220–7.

65. Norton TM, Cox S, Nelson SE, et al. Phamacokinetics of Tramadol and O-desmethyltramadol in loggerhead sea turtles (Caretta caretta). J Zoo Wildl Med 2015;46: 262–5.

66. Giorgi M, Salvadori M, De Vito V, et al. Pharmacokinetic/pharmacodynamic assessments of 10 mg/kg tramadol intramuscular injection in yellow-bellied slider turtles (Trachemys scripta scripta). J Vet Pharmacol Ther 2015;38:488–96.

67. Giorgi T, Rota S, Lee HK, et al. The pharmacokinetics and pharmacodynamics of a single intramuscular injection of tapentadol in yellow-bellied sliders (Trachemys scripta scripta). Proc Assoc Reptile Amphibian Vets 2014;58.

68. Williams CJA, James LE, Bertelsen MF, et al. Tachycardia in response to remote capsaicin injection as a model for nociception in the ball python (Python regius). Vet Anaesth Analg 2016;43:429–34.

69. Kinney M, Johnson SM, Sladky KK. Behavioral evaluation of red-eared slider turtles (Trachemys scripta) administered either morphine or butorphanol following unilateral gonadectomy. J Herpetol Med Surg 2011;21:54–62.

70. Scognamillo-Szabo MVR, Santos ALQ, Olegario MMM, et al. Acupuncture for locomotor disabilities in a South American red-footed tortoise (Geochelone carbonaria)—a case report. Acupunct Med 2008;26:243–7.

Pain in Birds
The Anatomical and Physiological Basis

Jamie M. Douglas, DVM, MS,
David Sanchez-Migallon Guzman, LV, MS, DECZM (Avian, Small Mammal), DACZM,
Joanne R. Paul-Murphy, DVM, DACZM, DACAW*

KEYWORDS

- Avian • Pain • Nociception • CNS • PNS

KEY POINTS

- Three types of nociceptors have been identified in the avian peripheral nervous system: high-threshold mechanothermal nociceptors, mechanical nociceptors, and thermal nociceptors.
- The C and Aδ nociceptor axons are located outside of the spinal cord at the dorsal root ganglia, where they bifurcate into peripheral and central branches, terminating at the nociceptors and the dorsal horn of the spinal cord respectively.
- The spinothalamic tract is the most significant sensory pathway for transmission of nociceptive signals including pain, temperature, and light touch, whereas the propriospinal tract is responsible for segmental reflexes.
- Pathway tracing and behavioral studies determined that visual, auditory, and somatosensory input goes from the thalamus to the striatal region in the avian brain, regions that carry out the same type of sensory information processing that is performed by the mammalian neocortex.
- Opioid receptors and related endorphin systems in normal physiologic functions are complex and also modulate pain. Information regarding distribution and structure of opioid receptors indicates differences among species.

INTRODUCTION

As defined by the International Association for the Study of Pain, pain is an unpleasant sensory and emotional experience associated with actual or potential tissue damage.[1] The emotional aspect of pain makes the sensation different from the classic senses, which are primarily informative in nature. The emotional aspect of pain also is difficult to measure in animals because they cannot verbally describe their discomfort. The

Disclosure Statement: The authors have nothing to disclose.
Department of Medicine and Epidemiology, School of Veterinary Medicine, University of California, Davis, 1 Garrod Drive, Davis, CA 95616, USA
* Corresponding author.
E-mail address: paulmurphy@ucdavis.edu

communication barrier between veterinarians and animals leaves practitioners to rely on behavioral observations to determine the presence of pain in their patients. For bird patients, assessment of pain can be particularly challenging. Avian species are predisposed to disguising pain, a survival mechanism that prevents unwanted attention from predators[2] and masks inferiority in instances of interspecific and intraspecific competition.[3] Instead, nociception, a process defined as the detection of noxious events by specialized peripheral sensory neurons found in the skin, muscle, joints, bone, and viscera of all vertebrates,[1,4] can be measured indirectly. Nociception generates a variety of physiologic and behavioral responses.[5]

Much of the information related to avian pain has been extrapolated from mammals, although significant avian-focused research has been published that illustrates anatomic and physiologic differences (**Fig. 1**). Despite some differences, birds possess the neurologic components necessary to respond to painful stimuli and they likely perceive pain in a manner similar to mammals.

PERIPHERAL NERVOUS SYSTEM

Noxious stimuli, events that damage or threaten damage to tissues,[1] are initially detected and encoded via nociceptors present in the avian peripheral nervous system (PNS). Largely, nociceptors are nonselective, gated cation channels, opening or closing in response to temperature, chemical ligands, or mechanical shearing forces.[6] When activated, nociceptors lead to a local depolarization of the terminal to initiate a conducted action potential. The nociceptors are associated with primary afferent nerve fibers. C fibers are the majority of the nerve fibers found in birds and are responsible for slow, diffuse pain that caters to a more diffuse, generalized pain sensation.[7] In contrast, the Aδ fibers are largely responsible for sharp, momentary pain and provide the precise localization of noxious stimuli.[7] C-type axons in birds have a conduction velocity of 0.3 m/s to 1 m/s, in contrast to a conduction velocity of 5 m/s to 40 m/s in the avian Aδ-type axons.[8] Slower conduction speeds in avian nerve fibers compared with the mammalian fibers are explained by smaller diameters and thinner myelin sheaths (when present).[9] Prolonged firing of C-fiber nociceptors in mammals causes release of glutamate, and this is assumed to be similar in birds. Glutamate then acts at N-methyl-D-aspartate receptors in the spinal cord and can lead to central sensitization.[10]

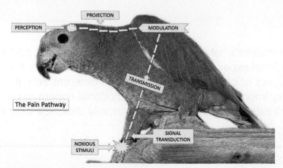

Fig. 1. Schematic illustration of the ascending pain pathway. A noxious stimulus at the periphery causes signal transduction at the nociceptor. The signal is transmitted along peripheral sensory axons to the cell body in the dorsal root ganglion, which then relays the signal to the dorsal horn of the spinal cord for processing, modulation, and projection to the brain along ascending spinal tracts. When nociceptive signals reach the brain, they are modulated and processed for cognitive and emotional perception. (*Courtesy of* Jamie M. Douglas, DVM, MS, Sacramento, CA.)

Three types of nociceptors have been identified in the avian PNS: high-threshold mechanothermal nociceptors, mechanical nociceptors, and thermal nociceptors.[11,12] The high-threshold mechanothermal nociceptors present in birds are polymodal. They respond to elevated temperatures (those above 104F), mechanical shearing, and chemical insult.[6] Avian high-threshold mechanothermal nociceptors are comparable to the C fibers present in mammals, conveying information to the central nervous system (CNS) slowly via unmyelinated axons.[1] Avian high-threshold mechanothermal nociceptors have been identified in the feathered skin of pigeons,[13] beak skin of geese,[14] and skin[15,16] and trigeminal mucosa[17] of chickens. Increasing the magnitude of noxious stimulus results in an increase in the number of high-threshold mechanothermal nociceptors activated, a result of the nociceptor's small receptive field. Differing from the high-threshold mechanoreceptor, birds also possess mechanical nociceptors. Avian mechanical nociceptors have axons and receptive fields of variable size[18] and have been identified in the skin of chickens[19] and geese.[14] Because the avian mechanoreceptors vary in size, mechanical nociceptors with small receptive fields are comparable to mammalian C fibers, whereas mechanical nociceptors with large receptive fields are similar to mammalian Aδ fibers. Thermal nociceptors are the third group of avian nociceptors, first identified in the chicken[11] and the pigeon.[13] Avian thermal nociceptors also have variable receptive fields and axon sizes. Avian thermal nociceptors are also distinct from the mammalian thermal nociceptors in that they are characterized as having a higher tolerance to heat and a decreased sensitivity to cold. In pigeons, 2 types of thermal nociceptors were found in the skin: 1 cold receptor that showed increased activity at low skin temperatures and 1 warm receptor that was excited by moderate heating.[13] This is not unexpected because the body and skin temperatures of birds are higher than in mammals. When comparing the physiologic responses of thermal nociceptors found in the chicken with those found in mammals, however, discharge patterns and receptive field size are similar.[19] Some nociceptors are also activated by specific chemicals. Birds are behaviorally insensitive to capsaicin, a potent irritant in mammals that leads to depletion of substance P at afferent terminals.[20] Birds, however, do demonstrate physiologic sensitivity to capsaicin.[21,22] Birds' inability to appreciate capsaicin as an irritant is thought to be an evolutionarily conserved trait.[23]

Other relevant anatomic features of the PNS in birds are the brachial plexus and lumbosacral plexuses. The anatomy of the avian brachial plexus has been studied in chickens,[24] mallard ducks (Anas platyrhynchos),[25] merlins (Falco columbarius),[26] and blue-fronted Amazon parrots (Amazona aestiva)[27] (Fig. 2). Customarily, the avian brachial plexus is composed of sympathetic nerve fibers with ventral branches of 3 to 5 nerves in 2 trunks, the accessory brachial and brachial.[28] The accessory brachial trunk is absent, however, in some avian species, such as the ostrich (Struthio camelus).[29] The complex anatomy of the brachial plexus has resulted in mixed success of regional anesthesia in birds,[24,25,30] with visualization, palpation, and blocking of the proximal brachial plexus hindered partially by the pectoral muscles.[27] There are 3 nerve plexuses in the lumbosacral region (lumbar, ischiatic, and pudendal). These nerve roots lie embedded in the foveae of the synsacrum and surrounded by the kidneys. All 3 plexuses are connected to the sympathetic chain.[28] Despite these differences in the lumbosacral region, sciatic-femoral nerve block has been successfully employed in peregrine falcons (Falco peregrinus).[31]

CENTRAL NERVOUS SYSTEM

A notable relevant difference in the avian spinal cord is its lack of cauda equina, with the avian spinal cord running the entire length of the vertebral canal.[6,32] The vertebrae

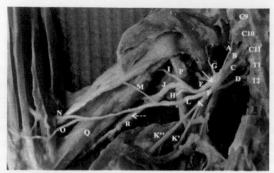

Fig. 2. Macrophotography of origin and distribution of brachial plexus in blue-fronted Amazon parrot (*Amazona aestiva*). This image demonstrates the anatomic complexity of the avian brachial plexus. The ventral branches of the spinal nerves C9 and C10 (trunk 1), C10 and C11 (trunk 2), C11 and T1 (trunk 3), and T1 and L2 (trunk 4) forms a common trunk (*arrow*), subdivided into dorsal and ventral cord. The supracoracoid, anconeal, axillary, radial nerves and their muscular branch (*dashed arrow*), pectoral trunk, and its cranial and caudal pectoral nerves, medianoulnar nerve, bicipital nerve, and median nerve and ulnar nerve, besides the caudal scapulohumeral muscles, humeral triceps, and scapular triceps. A, trunk 1; B, trunk 2; C, trunk 3; D, trunk 4; E, dorsal cord of trunk 4; F, ventral cord of trunk 4; G, supracoracoid nerve; H, anconeal nerve; I, axillary nerve; J, radial nerve; K, pectoral trunk; K', cranial pectoral trunk nerves; K", caudal pectoral trunk nerves; L, meadianoulnar nerve; M, bicipital nerve; N, median nerve; O, ulnar nerve; P, scapulohumeral muscles; Q, humeral triceps; R, scapular triceps. (*Data from* Silva RMNd, Figueiredo PdO, Santana MI. Formação e distribuição do plexo braquial em papagaios verdadeiros Amazona aestiva, linnaeus, 1758. Ciência Animal Brasileira 2015;16[3]:468; with permission.)

of birds are generally fused and their spinal nerves travel through the intervertebral foramina in a lateral direction (contrasting their caudal direction of travel in mammals). Most spinal nerves share numbers with the vertebrae just caudal to where they exit the spinal cord, although the last cervical spinal nerve exits the spinal canal caudal to the final cervical vertebrae and creates one more cervical spinal nerve than there are vertebrae.[6] The avian spinal cord is enlarged in both the cervical and lumbosacral regions of birds, corresponding to location of the brachial and lumbosacral plexuses respectively. Enlargement of the cervical spinal cord is more easily appreciated in birds that can fly.[32] The fusion of the spinal vertebrae in the pelvic region of birds is known as the synsacrum, where enlargement of the spinal canal and dorsally located splitting of the spinal cord forms a sinus. Housed within this sinus is the glycogen body, a collection of neuroglial cells that form a gelatinous, oval-shaped column unique to the avian spinal cord.[32] The meninges of birds consist of 3 layers: dura mater, arachnoid mater, and pia mater, providing protection and nutrients and creating a space in the spinal canal for cerebrospinal fluid.[6] Due to their unique anatomy of the avian spinal column (eg, fused vertebrae and lack of cauda equina), epidural anesthesia is not recommended in birds.

Overall, the anatomic arrangement of the avian spinal cord is similar to that of mammals. The somata of the C and Aδ nociceptor axons are located outside the spinal cord at the dorsal root ganglia, where they bifurcate into peripheral and central branches,[33] terminating at the nociceptors and the dorsal horn of the spinal cord respectively.[34] Spinal tracts form the outer white matter and the central butterfly-shaped area of gray matter of the spinal column, which receives information from peripheral receptors, including nociceptors. In addition, birds have marginal nuclei that surround the outer margins of the area of gray matter and these nuclei appear to be ventral commissural neurons that project information from one side of the cord to the other and, like mammals, may represent multisynaptic neurons that transmit nonlocalizing pain fibers up and down the spinal cord.[35]

The dorsal column nuclei are the predominant ascending pathway for tactile receptor transmission to the thalamus while also transmitting information from noxious stimulation of visceral and large cutaneous areas.[36] The fibers in the lateral spinothalamic tract are concerned with pain, synapsing in the substantia gelatinosa in the dorsal horn, decussating (intersecting), and then ascending in the lateral column of the spinal cord and brainstem to the thalamus. The spinothalamic tract is the most significant for transmission of nociceptive signals including pain, temperature, and light touch, although the propriospinal tract is responsible for segmental reflexes.[32] The propriospinal system involves short polysynaptic fibers that ascend the spinal cord to the reticular formation and delivers vague sensations of pain that are nonlocalized.[33,37]

The dorsal root ganglia are lateral to each segment of the spinal cord and contain the cell bodies of sensory neurons, including those activated by noxious stimuli. Peripheral nerves, including the central branches of C and Aδ nociceptor axons, transmit impulses and via the dorsal roots terminate primarily at the dorsal horn of the spinal cord.[34] In birds, primary afferent terminations in the dorsal horn can extend over several spinal segments and are not necessarily densest at the level of entry of the dorsal root fibers.[38] The cellular organization of the dorsal horn of the avian spinal cord varies between species. Some avian species, including pigeons and passerines, have a laminar organization of the dorsal horn similar to mammals. Most avian species are similar to the chicken, however, in which some of the laminae are side by side rather than in dorsoventral order.[39]

During nociceptive processing, a cascade of events takes place that play a role in the experience of pain. These events trigger highly variable regions of the brain in humans and because it is not a static or stand-alone entity has been termed, *the pain matrix*. The pain matrix refers to the substrate that is significantly and actively modulated by a variety of regions and receptors in the brain, dependent on the precise interplay of factors contributing to an individual person's perception of pain.[40] It has been well established that mammals possess areas in the brain required for the conscious perception of aversive elements associated with pain and birds likely have similar conscious experiences of the negative affective components of pain.[41] Evolutionary developmental studies often use the chicken embryo to study phylogenetic conservation and differentiation of brain structures between mammals and birds.[42] Both classes have a large cerebrum that makes up most of the brain, which is subdivided into pallial and subpallial regions (**Fig. 3**). The organization of the subpallium is similar between mammals and birds. The thalamus is located in the subpallial region of birds and is the central area of subcortical neural processing. It is the relay station for visual, auditory and somatosensory information. Pathway tracing and behavioral studies determined that visual, auditory, and somatosensory input goes from the thalamus to the striatal region in the avian brain, regions that carry out the same type of sensory information processing that is performed by the mammalian neocortex.[43] Despite that birds do not have an anatomically distinct cortex, both avian and mammalian forebrains show similarities in connectivity and function down to the cellular level.[44] The cerebral cortex (neocortex) is unique to mammals and occupies much of their dorsal telencephalon (pallium) and is characterized by a unique laminar structure where similar types of neurons are loosely arranged and form parallel layers. The avian pallium, in contrast, is not laminar and is histologically distinct from the mammalian pallium. Even with these dissimilarities, many regions of the avian pallium

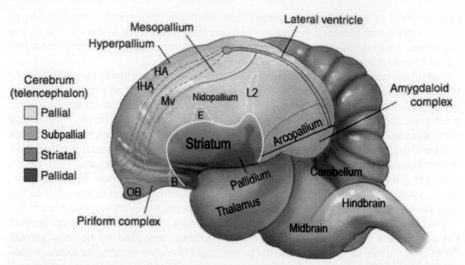

Fig. 3. Illustration of the songbird brain using anatomic terminology from the Avian Brain Nomenclature Forum. Major regions of the pallium (forebrain) include hyperpallium, mesopallium, nidopallium, arcopallium, and amygdaloid complex. B, basorostralis; E, entopallium; HA, hyperpallium apicale; IHA, interstitial hyperpallium apicale; L2, field L2; Mv, mesopallium ventral; OB, olfactory bulb. (*Modified from* Jarvis ED, Gunturkun O, Bruce L, et al. Avian brains and a new understanding of vertebrate brain evolution. Nat Rev Neurosci 2005;6[2]:154; with permission.)

remain homologous to the mammalian neocortex in function, each playing a role in cognitive and behavioral processing.[45–47] The structures of the brain involved in the complex affective processing of pain signals, however, are also those involved in the processing of other forms of complex information, including analysis of emotions unrelated to pain. It is because of this complex neural network that localization of the specific site of pain perception in the CNS of animals, including birds, has not yet occurred[28]; therefore, matching distinct areas of true homology of brain structures between mammals and birds continues to be a challenge and has been questioned by some investigators.

The development and implementation of functional neuroimaging have allowed minimally invasive examination of changes in the metabolic function of regions in the human brain during the experience of pain. Early studies of the functional localization of pain perception in the human brain assessed regional cerebral blood flow PET in association with pain stimulation.[48] A meta-analysis of human brain activation by pain using neuroimaging and regional cerebral blood flow studies concluded that brain regions, including the thalamus and regions of the cerebral cortex (including the insula and anterior cingulate cortex), have a significant likelihood of activation regardless of the type of noxious stimuli.[49] An unpublished avian study used the radioligand 18-fluroro-2-deoxy-D-glucose (FDG) to study regional cerebral glucose metabolism in the brain of anesthetized parrots experiencing pain from experimentally induced, temporary arthritis. Regional cerebral glucose metabolism under normal conditions was compared with its metabolism associated with the painful condition.[50] This study identified areas of the parrot cerebrum, including the nidopallium, associated with central processing of a persistent painful stimulus (**Fig. 4**). These findings provide supportive evidence that pain is a cognitive process for birds, much like it is in humans, and that pain increases metabolism in an area of the avian brain possibly rich in opioid

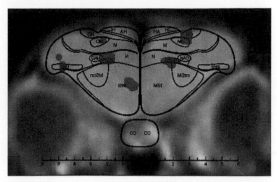

Fig. 4. Statistical parametric map (red) showing regions of significantly increased glucose metabolism associated with pain, overlaid on a scaled budgerigar atlas, and a Hispaniolan MRI template (grayscale). Four Hispaniolan parrots (*Amazona ventralis*) were scanned using microPET with FDG, 1 mCi administered intravenously. Experimental unilateral temporary inflammatory arthritis of the tarsal joint was used to model a painful condition. Parrots were imaged twice under anesthesia (3%–5% isoflurane in 100% oxygen) over 46 to 96 minutes after FDG injection in both nonarthritic and experimentally induced acute inflammatory arthritis conditions. Voxel-wise paired t-tests were thresholded at $P_{uncorrected}$ <.05 and random field theory was used to identify clusters (red) corrected for multiple comparisons at P<.05. The statistical map illustrates regions with increased whole brain normalized radioactivity, indicative of glucose metabolism, in experimental treatment verses control conditions. Map includes areas of the nidopallium (N), medial striatum (MSt), and oval nucleus of the mesopallium (MO), areas rich in endogenous opioid receptors and thought to be neurochemically and functionally similar to the mammalian prefrontal cortex. Bas, nucleus basorostralis; HD, hyperpallium densocellulare; M, mesopallium; MStm, magnocellular nucleus of medial striatum; NAO, oval nucleus of the anterior nidopallium; NAOm, medial oval nucleus of the anterior nidopallium.

receptors (**Fig. 5**). The application of microPET imaging techniques has been used to study opioid activity in other species and is an invaluable tool for future studies of physiologic changes in the CNS of birds during pain and the treatment of pain with pharmacologic agents.

Once nociceptive information is transmitted to the CNS of birds, the endogenous opioid system plays a crucial role in how that information is modulated. The endogenous opioid system functions in central processing of nociceptive information, with endogenous opioids (such as β-endorphin and enkephalin) binding to opioid receptors to inhibit pain.[51] In the avian brain, μ-opioid, κ-opioid, and δ-opioid receptors have been identified and mapped in the forebrain and midbrain of several avian species.[52–55] Spinal distribution of the μ-opioid and δ-opioid receptors has been examined using immunohistochemistry in the chicken.[56] The supraspinal distribution of μ, δ, and κ receptors has been described in the pigeon and the chicken using specific radiomarked ligands and autoradiographic receptor binding techniques.[53,54,57,58] In the pigeon forebrain, the κ receptor was the most abundant of the 3 classic opioid receptors; however, no relative predominance was noticed in the midbrain, similar to mammalian species.[53] In the chicken forebrain and midbrain, μ receptors were most prevalent and are detectable in chick embryos at 10 days of age.[54,59] Studies in a passerine species (dark-eyed junco [*Junco hyemalis*]) describe the autoradiographic distribution of μ-opioid, κ-opioid, and δ-opioid receptors in hypothalamic and vocal control regions.[60]

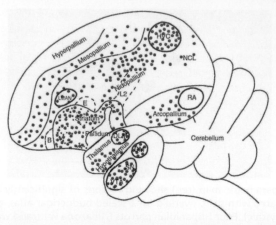

Fig. 5. A schematic representation of a songbird brain (sagittal view). Sketch shows distribution of κ-opioid receptors (*red dots*) and μ-opioid receptors (*blue dots*) as determined by studies of the song control system. These receptors are distributed across the nidopallium, striatum, VTA, and various nuclei, which correlate to centers of the brain for pleasure, reward, and song and are thought to correlate with release of endogenous opioids. Centers of the brain for pain or pathways for the avian pain matrix have not yet been determined, although the role of opioid receptors in normal physiologic functions is complex and includes endogenous response to pain, neuroendocrine functions, immunologic function, gastrointestinal function, cardiovascular function, pulmonary function, and cognition. B, basolateralis; DM, dorsal medial nucleus of the midbrain; DLM, dorsal lateral nucleus of the dorsomedial thalamus; E, entopallium; HVC, higher vocal center; L2, field L2; LMAN, lateral magnocellular nucleus of the anterior nidopallium; NCL, nidopallium caudolaterale; RA, robust nucleus of the arcopallium; SN, substantia nigra; VTA, ventral tegmental. (*Modified from* Emery NJ, Clayton NS. Do birds have the capacity for fun? Curr Biol 2015;25[1]:R18; with permission.)

Newer techniques, such as reverse transcriptase polymerase chain reaction and quantitative real-time polymerase chain reaction, have been applied to the zebra finch (*Taeniopygia guttata*) brain to study opioid receptors associated with song control, revealing higher levels of μ-opioid receptor mRNA compared with δ-opioid receptor mRNA in areas of the brain, such as the nidopallium.[61] In a recent presentation at a scientific meeting, the structure and expression of the μ-opioid, δ-opioid, and κ-opioid receptor genes in spinal, supraspinal, and peripheral tissues of a single peregrine falcon, a single snowy owl (*Bubo scandiacus*), and a single blue-fronted Amazon parrot were presented.[62] It has been frequently hypothesized that the variability of opioid effects observed between different avian species could be at least partially explained by differences not only in receptor distribution and density[53,63] but also in the receptor structure itself.[62] The role of opioid receptors and related endorphin systems in normal physiologic functions is complex and includes endogenous response to pain; however, opioid receptors are also associated with neuroendocrine functions, regulation of immunologic function, gastrointestinal function, cardiovascular function, pulmonary function, and cognition (**Fig. 5**). Information about the organization, structure, and function of opioid receptors in birds deserves further research.

γ-Aminobutyric acid (GABA) is the primary inhibitory neurotransmitter in the mammalian CNS, holding similar importance in avian species.[64] The GABA receptors are abundantly and heterogeneously distributed in the forebrain and midbrain of birds.[64] When the α, β, and γ subunits are present at the GABA$_A$ receptor, the receptor can become a binding site for benzodiazepines. In pigeons, $GABA_A$ receptors are more abundant in the brain than $GABA_B$ receptors, with γ-modified $GABA_A$ (benzodiazepine receptors) densely populated in the pallium.[65] The γ-modified $GABA_A$ receptor is important for its role in sedation, muscle relaxation, and anxiety.[66] Alongside GABA receptors, 2 cannabinoid receptors, cannabinoid$_1$ (CB_1) and cannabinoid$_2$ (CB_2), and 2 endogenous cannabinoids, anandamide and 2-arachidonylglycerol (2-AG), have been identified in mammals.[67] Research has shown that birds also possess CB_1 receptors in their CNS, evidenced in zebra finches,[68] chickens,[69] black-capped chickadees (Poecile atricapilla),[70] and budgerigars (Melopsittacus undulatus).[71] CB_2-like proteins have been described in the CNS of chick embryos[72] but are absent in the adult budgerigar brain.[71] Recent research has reported hyperphagia after both CB_1 and CB_2 agonism in neonatal layer-type chicks,[73] with endogenous nitrous oxide,[74] glutamate,[75] and $GABA$[76] amplifying the increased food intake cause by cannabinoids. Endogenous CB_2-AG was negatively correlated with fat mass in dark-eyed juncos whereas anandamide had no influence.[77] Although the endocannabinoid system can provide analgesia in mammals,[78–80] this function has not yet been explored in avian species.

PERIPHERAL AND CENTRAL SENSITIZATION

Pain is not only a nociceptive event. Peripheral sensitization is an increased response to an afferent stimulus from the nociceptors.[81] Sensitization of the mammalian PNS occurs once tissue damage results in lowering of pH and release of inflammatory mediators, 2 events that C fibers are sensitive to.[82] Inflammatory mediators released during peripheral sensitization include H^+, K^+, and prostaglandins (from damaged cells); bradykinin (from plasma); serotonin (from platelets); histamine (from mast cells); and cytokines (from macrophages).[6] In birds, storage and release of serotonin have been evidenced in duck[83] and chicken[84] thrombocytes, functional homologs of the mammalian platelet.[85] Modulation of inflammatory pain in the periphery can result in elevation of cyclooxygenase-2 levels at both the periphery and spinal cord.[86] Cyclooxygenase, or prostaglandin-endoperoxide synthase, metabolizes arachidonic acid into prostaglandins, involved in various aspects of the inflammatory response, including fever, hyperalgesia, and increased vascular permeability.[87] Cyclooxygenase expression has been demonstrated in chickens,[88–90] quail,[91] and ostrich,[92] with nonsteroidal anti-inflammatory drugs effective for pain management through nonselective cyclooxygenase inhibition in a variety of avian species.[93–95] The prostaglandins function in both promotion and resolution of inflammation,[96] with small-diameter nociceptor fibers (C fibers) of both mammals and birds sensitized to thermal and mechanical stimulation in the presence of these eicosanoids.[97,98] Additionally, prostaglandins have been shown to lower the threshold of activation of sensory neurons by activating nonselective cation channels.[99] Similarly, inflammatory mediator substance P also sensitizes avian C-fiber endings.[100] Substance P is released from sensory neurons in a dose-dependent manner after prostaglandin E_2 exposure enhances influx of calcium across neuronal cell membranes. The inward flux of calcium into sensory neurons causes release of substance P and cellular fluid, which is responsible for vasodilation, edema, and further activation and sensitization of the avian nociceptor.[15,98]

Central sensitization, in contrast to peripheral sensitization, occurs at dorsal horn neurons. As nociceptor activity increases, the threshold required to activate the dorsal horn neurons is decreased. The prolonged excitability of dorsal horn neurons results in recruitment of additional nerves and increased efficacy of nociceptive afferents.[101,102]

Characterization of both peripheral and central sensitization includes evidence of pain response at lower stimulus level, hastened response to noxious stimuli, prolonged response to noxious stimuli, increased magnitude of noxious stimulus, and spread of pain to uninjured tissues. Nociceptors' heightened response to inflammatory mediators can eventually reverse over time; however, chronic pain left untreated in any animal often results in maladaptation of the pain response. It can result include the development of hyperalgesia, a state of increased sensitivity to painful stimuli, and allodynia, a state in which innocuous items elicit a nociceptive response. Birds experiencing chronic pain may also display abnormal behaviors, a maladaptation that is often irreversible.[12] Research into chronic pain and maladaptive responses in avian species continues to be important to improve identification and management of pain in birds. The future of avian pain research needs to include understanding how the avian brain responds to acute pain and pain across time.

REFERENCES

1. Council NR. Recognition and alleviation of pain in laboratory animals, vol. 1. Washington, DC: National Academies Press; 2010.
2. Livingston A. Physiological basis for pain perception in animals. Vet Anaesth Analg 1994;21(2):73–7.
3. Svärdson G. Competition and habitat selection in birds. Oikos 1949;1(2): 157–74.
4. Dubin AE, Patapoutian A. Nociceptors: the sensors of the pain pathway. J Clin Invest 2010;120(11):3760–72.
5. Council NR. Definition of pain and distress and reporting requirements for laboratory animals: proceedings of the workshop held June 22, 2000. Washington, DC: The National Academies Press; 2000.
6. Whiteside DP. Analgesia. In: West G, Heard DJ, Caulkett N, editors. Zoo animal and wildlife immobilization and anesthesia. 2nd edition. Ames (IA): Blackwell Publishing; 2014. p. 83–108.
7. Giordano J. The neurobiology of pain. In: Weiner RS, editor. Pain management: a practical guide for clinicians. 6th edition. Boca Raton (FL): CRC press LLC; 2002. p. 1089–100.
8. Wild JM. The avian somatosensory system: a comparative view. In: Scanes CH, editor. Sturkie's Avian physiology. 6th edition. San Diego (CA): Academic Press; 2015. p. 55–69.
9. Necker R, Meinecke CC. Conduction velocities and fiber diameters in a cutaneous nerve of the pigeon. J Comp Physiol A 1984;154(6):817–24.
10. Bennett GJ. Update on the neurophysiology of pain transmission and modulation. J Pain Symptom Manage 2000;19(1):2–6.
11. Gentle MJ. Pain in birds. Anim Welfare 1992;1(4):235–47.
12. Paul-Murphy J, Hawkins MG. Bird-specific considerations: recognizing pain behavior in pet Birds. In: Gaynor JS, Muir WW III, editors. Handbook of veterinary pain management. 3rd edition. St Louis (MO): Elsevier Mosby; 2015. p. 536–54.
13. Necker R, Reiner B. Temperature-sensitive mechanoreceptors, thermoreceptors and heat nociceptors in the feathered skin of pigeons. J Comp Physiol A 1980; 135(3):201–7.
14. Gottschaldt KM, Fruhstorfer H, Schmidt W, et al. Thermosensitivity and its possible fine-structural basis in mechanoreceptors in the beak skin of geese. J Comp Neurol 1982;205(3):219–45.

15. Gentle MJ, Jones RB, Woolley SC. Physiological changes during tonic immobility in Gallus gallus var domesticus. Physiol Behav 1989;46(5):843–7.
16. Gentle MJ, Tilston V, McKeegan DE. Mechanothermal nociceptors in the scaly skin of the chicken leg. Neuroscience 2001;106(3):643–52.
17. McKeegan DE. Mechano-chemical nociceptors in the avian trigeminal mucosa. Brain Res Brain Res Rev 2004;46(2):146–54.
18. Gentle MJ, Hunter LN. Physiological and behavioural responses associated with feather removal in Gallus gallus var domesticus. Res Vet Sci 1991;50(1):95–101.
19. Holloway JA, Trouth CO, Wright LE, et al. Cutaneous receptive field characteristics of primary afferents and dorsal horn cells in the avian (Gallus domesticus). Exp Neurol 1980;68(3):477–88.
20. Szolcsányi J, Sann H, Pierau F-K. Nociception in pigeons is not impaired by capsaicin. Pain 1986;27(2):247–60.
21. Sann H, Harti G, Pierau FK, et al. Effect of capsaicin upon afferent and efferent mechanisms of nociception and temperature regulation in birds. Can J Physiol Pharmacol 1987;65(6):1347–54.
22. Harti G, Sharkey KA, Pierau FK. Effects of capsaicin in rat and pigeon on peripheral nerves containing substance P and calcitonin gene-related peptide. Cell Tissue Res 1989;256(3):465–74.
23. Kirifides ML. Calcium responses of chicken trigeminal ganglion neurons to methyl anthranilate and capsaicin. J Exp Biol 2004;207(5):715–22.
24. Figueiredo JP, Cruz ML, Mendes GM, et al. Assessment of brachial plexus blockade in chickens by an axillary approach. Vet Anaesth Analg 2008;35(6): 511–8.
25. Brenner DJ, Larsen RS, Dickinson PJ, et al. Development of an avian brachial plexus nerve block technique for perioperative analgesia in mallard ducks (Anas platyrhynchos). J Avian Med Surg 2010;24(1):24–34.
26. Cevik-Demirkan A. Anatomical structure of the brachial plexus in the merlin (Falco columbarius). Anat Histol Embryol 2014;43(1):31–5.
27. Silva RMNd, Figueiredo PdO, Santana MI. Formação e distribuição do plexo braquial em papagaios verdadeiros (Amazona aestiva, Linnaeus, 1758). Ciência Anim Brasileira 2015;16(3):464–73.
28. Bennett RA. Neurology. In: Ritchie BW, Harrison GJ, Harrison LR, editors. Avian medicine: principles and application. Lake Worth (FL): Wingers Pub; 1994. p. 723–45.
29. Pospieszny N, Pachulska P, Paździor K, et al. Nerves of thoracic limb of the ostrich (Struthio camelus L.). EJPAU 2009;12(4). Available at: http://www.ejpau.media.pl/volume12/issue4/art-08.html.
30. da Cunha AF, Strain GM, Rademacher N, et al. Palpation- and ultrasound-guided brachial plexus blockade in Hispaniolan Amazon parrots (Amazona ventralis). Vet Anaesth Analg 2013;40(1):96–102.
31. d'Ovidio D, Noviello E, Adami C. Nerve stimulator-guided sciatic-femoral nerve block in raptors undergoing surgical treatment of pododermatitis. Vet Anaesth Analg 2015;42(4):449–53.
32. Orosz SE, Antinoff N. Clinical avian neurology and neuroanatomy. In: Speers BL, editor. Current therapy in avian medicine and surgery. 1st edition. St Louis (MO): Elsevier; 2016. p. 363–77.
33. Necker R. The Somatosensory System, Functional Organization of the Spinal Cord. In: Whittow GC, editor. Sturkie's Avian physiology. 5th edition. San Diego (CA): Academic Press; 2000. p. 57–69, 71–81.

34. Wan Q, Pang SF. Segmental, coronal and subcellular distribution of 2-[125 I] io-
    domelatonin binding sites in the chicken spinal cord. Neurosci Lett 1994;180(2):
    253–6.
35. King AS, McLelland J. The Nervous System. Birds: their structure and function.
    2nd edition. Philadelphia: Bailliere Tindall; 1984. p. 240–1.
36. Wild JM. Avian somatosensory system: II. Ascending projections of the dorsal
    column and external cuneate nuclei in the pigeon. J Comp Neurol 1989;
    287(1):1–18.
37. Baumel J. Suspensory ligaments of nerves: an adaptation for protection of the
    avian spinal cord. Anat Histol Embryol 1985;14(1):1–5.
38. Gentle MJ, Hunter LN, Sterling RJ. Projections of ankle joint afferents to the spi-
    nal cord and brainstem of the chicken (Gallus g. domesticus). J Comp Neurol
    1995;361(4):669–80.
39. Wild JM, Krützfeldt NO, Altshuler DL. Trigeminal and spinal dorsal horn (dis)
    continuity and avian evolution. Brain Behav Evol 2010;76(1):11–9.
40. Bingel U, Tracey I. Imaging CNS modulation of pain in humans. Physiology
    (Bethesda) 2008;23(6):371–80.
41. Le Neindre P, Bernard E, Boissy A, et al. Animal consciousness. EFSA Support-
    ing Publications 2017;14(4).
42. Suzuki IK, Hirata T. Neocortical neurogenesis is not really "neo": a new evolu-
    tionary model derived from a comparative study of chick pallial development.
    Dev Growth Differ 2013;55(1):173–87.
43. Jarvis ED, Gunturkun O, Bruce L, et al. Avian brains and a new understanding of
    vertebrate brain evolution. Nat Rev Neurosci 2005;6(2):151–9.
44. Güntürkün O, Bugnyar T. Cognition without cortex. Trends Cogn Sci 2016;20(4):
    291–303.
45. Northcutt RG, Kaas JH. The emergence and evolution of mammalian neocortex.
    Trends Neurosci 1995;18(9):373–9.
46. Medina L, Reiner A. Do birds possess homologues of mammalian primary
    visual, somatosensory and motor cortices? Trends Neurosci 2000;23(1):1–12.
47. Jarvis ED. Evolution of the pallium in birds and reptiles. In: Binder MD,
    Hirokawa N, Windhorst U, et al, editors. Encyclopedia of neuroscience. Berlin:
    Springer-Verlag; 2009. p. 1390–400. Springer.
48. Xu X, Fukuyama H, Yazawa S, et al. Functional localization of pain perception in
    the human brain studied by PET. Neuroreport 1997;8(2):555–9.
49. Duerden EG, Albanese MC. Localization of pain-related brain activation: A
    meta-analysis of neuroimaging data. Hum Brain Mapp 2013;34(1):109–49.
50. Paul-Murphy J, Sladky KK, McCutcheon RA, et al. Using positron emission to-
    mography imaging of the parrot brain to study response to clinical pain. Paper
    presented at: 2005 Annual Conference of the Academy of Molecular Imaging.
    Orlando (FL), March 18–23, 2005.
51. Reiner A, Davis BM, Brecha NC, et al. The distribution of enkephalinlike immu-
    noreactivity in the telencephalon of the adult and developing domestic chicken.
    J Comp Neurol 1984;228(2):245–62.
52. Bardo MT, Bhatnagar RK, Gebhart GF, et al. Opiate receptor development in
    midbrain and forebrain of posthatch chicks. Brain Res 1982;255(4):668–73.
53. Reiner A, Brauth SE, Kitt CA, et al. Distribution of mu, delta, and kappa opiate
    receptor types in the forebrain and midbrain of pigeons. J Comp Neurol
    1989;280(3):359–82.
54. Csillag A, Bourne RC, Stewart MG. Distribution of mu, delta, and kappa
    opioid receptor binding sites in the brain of the one-day-old domestic chick

(*Gallus domesticus*): an in vitro quantitative autoradiographic study. J Comp Neurol 1990;302(3):543–51.

55. Deviche P, Cotter P, Gulledge CC. Identification, partial characterization, and hypothalamic distribution of κ, μ, and δ opioid receptors in a passerine songbird (*Junco hyemalis*). Brain Res 1993;614(1–2):220–6.

56. Kawate T, Sakamoto H, Yang C, et al. Immunohistochemical study of delta and mu opioid receptors on synaptic glomeruli with substance P-positive central terminals in chicken dorsal horn. Neurosci Res 2005;53(3):279–87.

57. Mansour A, Khachaturian H, Lewis ME, et al. Anatomy of CNS opioid receptors. Trends Neurosci 1988;11(7):308–14.

58. Csillag A, Bourne RC, Kalman M, et al. [3H]naloxone binding in the brain of the domestic chick (*Gallus domesticus*) determined by in vitro quantitative autoradiography. Brain Res 1989;479(2):391–6.

59. Hendrickson CM, Lin S. Opiate receptors in highly purified neuronal cell populations isolated in bulk from embryonic chick brain. Neuropharmacology 1980; 19(8):731–9.

60. Gulledge CC, Deviche P. Autoradiographic localization of opioid receptors in vocal control regions of a male passerine bird (*Junco hyemalis*). J Comp Neurol 1995;356(3):408–17.

61. Khurshid N, Agarwal V, Iyengar S. Expression of mu- and delta-opioid receptors in song control regions of adult male zebra finches (*Taenopygia guttata*). J Chem Neuroanat 2009;37(3):158–69.

62. Duhamelle A, Raiwet D, Langlois I, et al. Structure and expression of opioid receptor genes in the peregrine falcon (Falco peregrinus), the snowy owl (Bubo scandiacus) and the blue-fronted Amazon (Amazona aestiva). Paper presented at: ICARE 2017. Venice (Italy), March 25–29, 2017.

63. Emery NJ, Clayton NS. Do birds have the capacity for fun? Curr Biol 2015;25(1): R16–20.

64. Veenman CL, Reiner A. The distribution of GABA-containing perikarya, fibers, and terminals in the forebrain and midbrain of pigeons, with particular reference to the basal ganglia and its projection targets. J Comp Neurol 1994;339(2): 209–50.

65. Veenman CL, Albin RL, Richfield EK, et al. Distributions of GABAA, GABAB, and benzodiazepine receptors in the forebrain and midbrain of pigeons. J Comp Neurol 1994;344(2):161–89.

66. Fritschy JM, Panzanelli P. GABAA receptors and plasticity of inhibitory neurotransmission in the central nervous system. Eur J Neurosci 2014;39(11): 1845–65.

67. Piomelli D, Giuffrida A, Calignano A, et al. The endocannabinoid system as a target for therapeutic drugs. Trends Pharmacol Sci 2000;21(6):218–24.

68. Soderstrom K, Johnson F. CB1 cannabinoid receptor expression in brain regions associated with zebra finch song control. Brain Res 2000;857(1–2):151–7.

69. Fowler CJ, Borjesson M, Tiger G. Differences in the pharmacological properties of rat and chicken brain fatty acid amidohydrolase. Br J Pharmacol 2000;131(3): 498–504.

70. Shiflett MW, Rankin AZ, Tomaszycki ML, et al. Cannabinoid inhibition improves memory in food-storing birds, but with a cost. Proc Biol Sci 2004;271(1552): 2043–8.

71. Alonso-Ferrero ME, Paniagua MA, Mostany R, et al. Cannabinoid system in the budgerigar brain. Brain Res 2006;1087(1):105–13.

72. Fowler CJ, Nilsson O, Andersson M, et al. Pharmacological properties of cannabinoid receptors in the avian brain: similarity of rat and chicken cannabinoid1 receptor recognition sites and expression of cannabinoid2 receptor-like immunoreactivity in the embryonic chick brain. Pharmacol Toxicol 2001;88(4):213–22.

73. Alizadeh A, Zendehdel M, Babapour V, et al. Role of cannabinoidergic system on food intake in neonatal layer-type chicken. Vet Res Commun 2015;39(2): 151–7.

74. Hassanpour S, Zendehdel M, Babapour V, et al. Endocannabinoid and nitric oxide interaction mediates food intake in neonatal chicken. Br Poult Sci 2015; 56(4):443–51.

75. Keyshams N, Zendehdel M, Babapour V, et al. Cannabinoid-glutamate interactions in the regulation of food intake in neonatal layer- type chicks: role of glutamate NMDA and AMPA receptors. Vet Res Commun 2016;40(2):63–71.

76. Zendehdel M, Tirgari F, Shohre B, et al. Involvement of gaba and cannabinoid receptors in central food intake regulation in neonatal layer chicks: role of Cb1 and Gabaa receptors. Revista Brasileira de Ciência Avícola 2017;19(2): 221–30.

77. Ho JM, Bergeon Burns CM, Rendon NM, et al. Lipid signaling and fat storage in the dark-eyed junco. Gen Comp Endocrinol 2017;247:166–73.

78. Herzberg U, Eliav E, Bennett G, et al. The analgesic effects of R (+)-WIN 55,212–2 mesylate, a high affinity cannabinoid agonist, in a rat model of neuropathic pain. Neurosci Lett 1997;221(2):157–60.

79. Rice AS, Farquhar-Smith WP, Nagy I. Endocannabinoids and pain: spinal and peripheral analgesia in inflammation and neuropathy. Prostaglandins Leukot Essent Fatty Acids 2002;66(2–3):243–56.

80. Hohmann AG, Suplita RL, Bolton NM, et al. An endocannabinoid mechanism for stress-induced analgesia. Nature 2005;435(7045):1108–12.

81. Chapman CR, Casey K, Dubner R, et al. Pain measurement: an overview. Pain 1985;22(1):1–31.

82. Davidson S, Copits BA, Zhang J, et al. Human sensory neurons: Membrane properties and sensitization by inflammatory mediators. Pain 2014;155(9): 1861–70.

83. Stiller RA, Belamarich FA, Shepro D. Aggregation and release in thrombocytes of the duck. Am J Physiol 1975;229(1):206–10.

84. Bult H, Wechsung E, Houvenaghel A, et al. Prostanoids and hemostasis in chickens: anti-aggregating activity of prostaglandins E1 and E2, but not of prostacyclin and prostaglandin D2. Prostaglandins 1981;21(6):1045–58.

85. Claver JA, Quaglia AIE. Comparative morphology, development, and function of blood cells in nonmammalian vertebrates. J Exot Pet Med 2009;18(2):87–97.

86. Mitchell JA, Warner TD. Cyclo-oxygenase-2: pharmacology, physiology, biochemistry and relevance to NSAID therapy. Br J Pharmacol 1999;128(6): 1121–32.

87. Morteau O. Prostaglandins and inflammation: the cyclooxygenase controversy. In: Górski A, Krotkiewski H, Zimecki M, editors. Inflammation. Netherlands: Springer; 2001. p. 67–81.

88. Anhut H, Brune K, Frölich JC, et al. Prostaglandin D2 is the prevailing prostaglandin in the acute inflammatory exudate of urate arthritis in the chicken. Br J Pharmacol 1979;65(3):357–9.

89. Mathonnet M, Lalloue F, Danty E, et al. Cyclo-oxygenase 2 tissue distribution and developmental pattern of expression in the chicken. Clin Exp Pharmacol Physiol 2001;28(5–6):425–32.

90. Yamada S, Kawate T, Sakamoto H, et al. Cyclo-oxygenase-2-immunoreactive neurons in the lumbar dorsal horn in a chicken acute inflammation model. Anat Sci Int 2006;81(3):164–72.
91. Rodler D, Sinowatz F. Expression of prostaglandin-synthesizing enzymes (cyclooxygenase 1, cyclooxygenase 2) in the ovary of the quail (*Coturnix japonica*). Folia Biol (Praha) 2015;61:125–33.
92. Rodler D, Sinowatz F. Expression of prostaglandin synthesizing enzymes (cyclooxygenase 1 and cyclooxygenase 2) in the ovary of the ostrich (*Struthio camelus*). Acta Histochem 2015;117(1):69–75.
93. Danbury T, Weeks C, Chambers J, et al. Self-selection of the analgesic drug carprofen by lame broiler chickens. Vet Rec 2000;146(11):307–11.
94. Machin KL, Livingston A. Assessment of the analgesic effects of ketoprofen in ducks anesthetized with isoflurane. Am J Vet Res 2002;63(6):821–6.
95. Cole GA, Paul-Murphy J, Krugner-Higby L, et al. Analgesic effects of intramuscular administration of meloxicam in Hispaniolan parrots (*Amazona ventralis*) with experimentally induced arthritis. J Am Vet Med Assoc 2009;235(12):1436.
96. Ricciotti E, Fitzgerald GA. Prostaglandins and inflammation. Arterioscler Thromb Vasc Biol 2011;31(5):986–1000.
97. Martin HA, Basbaum AI, Kwiat GC, et al. Leukotriene and prostaglandin sensitization of cutaneous high-threshold C- and A-delta mechanonociceptors in the hairy skin of rat hindlimbs. Neuroscience 1987;22(2):651–9.
98. Nicol GD, Klingberg DK, Vasko MR. Prostaglandin E2 increases calcium conductance and stimulates release of substance P in avian sensory neurons. J Neurosci 1992;12(5):1917–27.
99. Meves H. The action of prostaglandins on ion channels. Curr Neuropharmacol 2006;4(1):41–57.
100. Zhai XY, Atsumi S. Large dorsal horn neurons which receive inputs from numerous substance P-like immunoreactive axon terminals in the laminae I and II of the chicken spinal cord. Neurosci Res 1997;28(2):147–54.
101. Campbell JN, Meyer RA. Mechanisms of neuropathic pain. Neuron 2006;52(1): 77–92.
102. Woolf CJ. Central sensitization: implications for the diagnosis and treatment of pain. Pain 2011;152(3 Suppl):S2–15.

Avian Ganglioneuritis in Clinical Practice

Giacomo Rossi, DVM, PhD, DECZM (Wildlife Population Health)[a],
Robert D. Dahlhausen, DVM, MS[b], Livio Galosi, DVM[a],
Susan E. Orosz, PhD, DVM, DABVP (Avian), DECZM (Avian)[c],*

KEYWORDS

- Avian ganglioneuritis • Avian bornavirus • Bornaviridae
- Proventricular dilatation disease

KEY POINTS

- Avian ganglioneuritis (AG) comprises one of the most intricate pathologies in avian medicine and is researched worldwide.
- Avian bornavirus (ABV) has been shown to be a causative agent of proventricular dilatation disease (AG/PDD) in birds.
- The avian Bornaviridae represent a genetically diverse group of viruses that are widely distributed in captive and wild populations around the world.

INTRODUCTION

Neuropathic gastric dilatation of psittacine birds was initially reported as a wasting disease in macaws imported into North America and Europe from Bolivia in the late 1970s.[1–8] Originally limited to macaw species (*Ara* spp.), the disease was later identified in other parrot species as well. One of the first reports was by Ridgway and Gallerstein in 1983 followed by the report of impaction, dilatation, and degeneration of the proventriculus in 16 large psittacine birds by Clark in 1984.[1,6] Originally called macaw wasting disease, the disease has also been referred to as macaw fading syndrome, myenteric ganglioneuritis, infiltrative splanchnic neuropathy, neuropathic gastric dilatation, and proventricular dilatation disease (PDD). The disease may be more appropriately termed avian myenteric ganglioneuritis, nonsuppurative ganglioneuritis, avian autoimmune ganglioneuritis, or simply, avian ganglioneuritis (AG).[9] These articulate the disease process better and remove the focus on the proventriculus. For this document, the newer term AG will be used synonymously with AG/PDD.

The authors have nothing to disclose.
[a] Animal Pathology Section, School of Biosciences and Veterinary Medicine, University of Camerino, Via Circonvallazione 93, 62024 Matelica, Italy; [b] Avian and Exotic Animal Medical Center and Veterinary Molecular Diagnostics, Inc, 5989 Meijer Drive, Suite 5, Milford, OH 45150, USA; [c] Bird and Exotic Pet Wellness Center, 5166 Monroe Street, Suite 306, Toledo, OH 43623, USA
* Corresponding author.
E-mail address: DrSusanOrosz@aol.com

AG/PDD has been described in more than 80 species of psittacine and nonpsitta-cine birds worldwide, both captive and in the wild.[10,11] African grey parrots (*Psittacus erithacus*), macaws (*Ara* species), Amazon parrots (*Amazona* species), and cockatoos (*Cacatua* species) are the most common psittacine species affected.[10] The disease is minimally represented in Quaker parrots (*Myiopsitta monachus*) and lovebird species (*Agapornis*).[9] Lesions suggestive of AG/PDD have also been described in canaries (*Serinus canaria*), the greenfinch (*Carduelis chloris*), long-wattled umbrella bird (*Ceph-alopterus penduliger*), a bearded barbet *(Lybius dubius)*, Canada geese (*Branta cana-densis*), toucans (Rhamphastidae), honey creepers (Drepanidinae), roseate spoonbill (*Platalea ajaja*), and a peregrine falcon (*Falco peregrines*).[12-15] AG/PDD is a progres-sive neurologic disease with a high case fatality rate once clinical signs are present.[16] The disease presents a serious threat to captive propagation and conservation efforts for endangered psittacines, such as the Spix macaw (*Cyanopsitta spixii*).

AVIAN GANGLIONEURITIS
Clinical Signs

Clinical signs are variable and depend on the host species involved, severity of dis-ease, distribution of lesions, and the organs affected or the nuclei of the nervous sys-tem that are impaired. These clinical signs vary from patient to patient. They often result from the parts of the central (CNS), peripheral (PNS), and/or autonomic nervous system that are affected by the pathologic process. Although often neurogenic in na-ture, signs are generally classified as gastrointestinal (GI) or CNS in character. Birds may exhibit only GI or neurologic signs or a combination of both. GI tract signs often reflect pathology of the terminal ganglia of the vagus nerve (cranial nerve [CN] X).

Myocarditis as a component of AG/PDD has been reported previously.[17] Lesions are more frequent and severe in the right side of the heart, which may reflect the higher density of nerves in this area. Additionally, parasympathetic innervation of the heart is partially controlled by the right vagus branch, which innervates the sinoatrial node. Dilatation of the right ventricle of the heart in affected birds has previously been described. Arrhythmias and alterations in blood pressure also may be observed. Car-diac lesions can result in acute death in otherwise clinically normal birds.

Signs Associated with the Nervous System

Particularly in New World species of parrots, clinical signs often relate to the vagus nerve. The vagus, also referred to as the pneumogastric nerve, is the autonomic ner-vous system's parasympathetic control of the heart and proximal digestive tract. It regulates homeostatic function of the proximal GI tract, pancreatic endocrine and exocrine function, hepatic glucose production, and heart rate. GI signs reflect varying degrees of dysfunction and neurogenic atrophy. These include delayed crop emptying and impaired GI tract transit, regurgitation, anorexia, dilatation, and sometimes impaction of the upper GI tract. Pyloric motility can be disturbed with severe alteration of gastric emptying and stasis.

The vagus nerve represents the preganglionic parasympathetic fibers from the dor-sal vagal nucleus of the medulla in the caudal brainstem. This nucleus occupies the medial portion of the floor of the fourth ventricle in mammals and consists of a column of cells that extend both rostrally and caudally in the medulla. It is found in a similar location in birds.[18] In mammals, the column consists of small-spindle shaped cells scattered among larger cells with a melanic pigment. The functional significance relating to the cell types is unclear. These cells have axons that give rise to the pregan-glionic parasympathetic fibers that travel to a variety of organs, including the proximal

GI tract, heart, and lungs. These preganglionic fibers will synapse in the wall of the organ in smaller collections of cell bodies, the terminal or myenteric ganglia. From there, the postganglionic parasympathetic fibers that arise from these terminal ganglia innervate the smooth muscle of the organs, including the heart, lungs, and GI tract from the esophagus to the transverse colon.[19] Some anatomists suggest that these visceral efferent neurons act as interneurons, as they may not have direct initiation of the smooth muscle activity to the digestive tract. They may, instead, modulate the intrinsic activity of the enteric plexus.[20] In some animal species, the intrinsic neural activity is strong and can maintain small intestinal peristalsis and colonic movement with the smooth muscle cells contracting rhythmically. In these species, the vagus appears to only modify this intrinsic activity.

The cells within the dorsal vagal nucleus are precisely arranged anatomically to provide innervation to a part or segment of an organ, including the GI tract, and this anatomic relationship can be observed clinically. For example, in some parrots only the motility of the crop has been affected, and in others, the stomach only. It would appear from the signs observed in parrots, that the vagus plays an important role in the mixing of GI contents in the stomach (proventriculus and ventriculus), as well as normal transit of foodstuffs. Based on the clinical signs observed with AG that often include severe changes in mixing of stomach contents, in parrots at least, the vagus nerve may play a major role for normal enteric peristalsis and retroperistalsis. This clinical observation differs from the suggestion of Tizard and colleagues[21] that the interstitial cells of Cajal (ICC) are altered by avian bornavirus (ABV), producing the symptoms observed.

Gut motility of the mammalian stomach is regulated by slow waves that are generated from the ICC that are found near the myenteric plexus. These cells are thought to pace the muscles to cause contraction. There are several of these pacemaker regions along the GI tract that result in distinct differences in the slow-wave frequency.[22] However, because the stomach of most birds lacks the longitudinal smooth muscle layer, they do not display the slow waves like in mammals. Dziuk and Duke[23] instead determined that gastric motility of birds was more complex than in mammals.

The stomach of birds is divided into various regions, which is distinct from the carnivorous mammalian stomach. In birds, there is a proximal glandular portion of the stomach, the proventriculus, that is linked to the more grinding portion, the gizzard or ventriculus, with a short isthmus or intermediate zone. The pyloric or distal portion of the stomach regulates the outflow of the contents of the gizzard to the duodenum. The glandular proventriculus secretes the gastric juices for digestion of foodstuffs. The gizzard is the site of gastric proteolysis and can also provide, depending on its anatomy of the species, mechanical digestion. In granivores, including chickens and turkeys, the muscles that do the grinding are prominent, whereas in parrots, that are frugivores, the muscles are more intermediate. This gizzard has reduced musculature in comparison with the granivores but more than found in carnivores.[24] The wall of the gizzard consists of 4 semiautonomous layers of smooth muscle that are derived from the circular smooth muscle layer and are asymmetrically arranged. They consist of the caudodorsal and cranioventral thick layers with craniodorsal and caudoventral thin layers. This anatomic arrangement provides the rotatory and crushing movements when the gizzard contracts.[24]

Our understanding of the motility of the stomach of birds is based on turkey and chicken models (granivores), which have a highly muscular ventriculus. Parrots (frugivores) have a reduced muscular stomach in comparison, but the mixing on fluoroscopy appears to be similar in normal parrots when compared with chickens (Orosz, personal observations, 1997). During the gastrointestinal cycle of birds, the thin muscles of the muscular stomach contract and the isthmus closes. The pylorus opens and the gastric contents flow into the duodenum. Next the duodenum contracts. This precipitates the relaxation of the isthmus and contraction of the thick muscles of the gizzard, producing grinding of contents and a rotatory movement of contents into the glandular stomach. Larger particles are retained in the gizzard longer for continued grinding.[24] Although initiation of the cycle is not dependent on the vagus nerve in satiated granivorous birds, in fasted birds, its denervation slows the rate of the gastrointestinal cycle and disrupts is normal synchronization. Chaplin and Duke[25] showed that the pacemaker for the gastrointestinal cycle appears to be in the isthmus. They found that destruction of the myenteric plexus in this area reduced contractions of the muscular stomach and the duodenum by 50%, even in granivorous birds, and simultaneously abolished the contractions of the glandular stomach. These physiology findings are similar to those observed using fluoroscopy to observe the alteration of mixing in parrots with the GI form of AG/PDD disease (Orosz, personal communication, 1997).

One hypothesis is that ABV with AG/PDD affects the ICC, thereby causing the changes observed with a flaccid stomach.[21] However, the previously mentioned studies suggest that the alteration of the myenteric plexus that is observed histopathologically would explain these clinical observations. ICCs are mesenchymally derived cells, belonging to the family of smooth muscle cells in which the activation of Kit signaling (c-Kit receptor, which is shaped by a CD117-specific antibody) is required for their development. In addition, the ICC cells of the chicken may be embryologically derived from neural tube cells. Morphologic studies have identified different phenotypic classes of ICC with different regulatory roles within the gut that contribute to both the regulation of excitation–contraction coupling and to connectivity between smooth muscle cells and the motor output of the enteric nervous system. ICC functions include (1) generation of electrical slow-wave activity in phasic regions of the GI tract, (2) coordination of pacemaker activity and active propagation of slow waves, (3) transduction of motor neural inputs from the enteric nervous system, (4) mechanosensation to stretch of GI muscles, and (5) setting the membrane potential gradient of gut smooth muscles. However, further in vivo studies are needed to support these proposed roles of ICC in the GI tract of birds and particularly parrots. ICC abnormalities or decreases in the number of ICCs has been reported in some GI tract diseases. However, understanding the nature of the interrelationship between ICC and the generation of gut motility disorders and the underlying mechanism for ICC loss is currently under investigation.

Additionally, ICCs have been grouped according to either their localization within the muscle layers (submuscular [ICC-SM], intramuscular [ICC-IM], myenteric [ICC-MY], and subserosal [ICC-SS]), their basic morphology (stellate and bipolar), or their primary function. These functions include pacemaker cells, cells that mediate neuromuscular neurotransmission and/or mechanoreceptor cells. ICCs in the smooth muscle of the esophagus, crop, and within the lower esophageal sphincter are of the ICC-IM subtype. They are in close contact with nerve terminals and make specific junctions (including nexuses) with smooth muscle cells.[26] There is no aggregation of ICC-IM around the myenteric plexus or at the submucosal border, as in the small and large intestines. In the proventriculus and gizzard, ICCs are more densely located in the corpus and antrum than in the fundus; the antrum contains both ICC-MY and ICC-IM networks, whereas in the fundus only ICC-IM cells are found.[27,28] Along the circumferential axis of the antrum, ICC-MY cells are distributed more densely in the greater curvature than in the lesser curvature.[27,28] Although these cells are intriguing in understanding normal physiologic function of peristalsis and retroperistalsis in birds, those functions in birds with AG/PDD lesions remain unclear. In studies performed by immunohistochemistry on ICC, no decrease has been observed in these ICC-SM and ICC-IM cells at the intramuscular level, in the area of the pylorus and/or in the proventricular antral area of AG/PDD-affected parrots (**Fig. 1**) (Rossi, personal communication, 2017).

Studies in the cat suggest that the dorsal vagal nucleus, in addition to its innervation and control of smooth muscle activity, is also the source of innervation to the glandular structures of the visceral mucosa. Based on this information, gastric acid secretion can be affected in some species of animals as well, and this may play a role in parrots.[19,20] Alteration of the normal release of the proteolytic enzymes and hydrochloric acid in the stomach and proximal small intestine affect digestion and absorption of foodstuffs. This may explain the symptoms observed in some birds affected by this disease. AG/PDD-affected parrots with proximal GI tract dysfunction have impaired ability to digest and absorb dietary nutrients, leading to loss of body weight, passage of undigested food material in the feces, and osmotically induced diarrhea (Orosz, personal observations over 33 years).

The vagus nerve is also a major constituent of the inflammatory reflex, a neural reflex that controls innate immune responses and inflammation during GI tract pathogen invasion and tissue injury.[29–31] Impairment of this reflex and reduced vagal stimulation of gastric acids impairs the natural resistance to bacterial overgrowth and leads to alterations in the intestinal microbiome. Overgrowth of pathogenic organisms, such as clostridial species and fungal organisms, particularly yeasts, including *Macrorhabdus ornithogaster*, often occur in affected parrots and other species.

In addition to the GI tract, signs can include those from the heart or the lungs, although linking respiratory signs to AG/PDD has not been documented to date. The vagus nerve innervates these organs through the dorsal vagal nucleus. It has been suggested the CN-X provides input to the carotid body to the heart, not the glossopharyngeal nerve (CN IX) in birds. Because it appears clinically that CN-X is affected by AG/PDD in a number of New World psittacines, then these findings support this anatomic observation.

In birds, the main trunk of the vagus travels down the neck alongside the jugular vein and does not give off any branches until it reaches the thorax. At the thoracic inlet, it

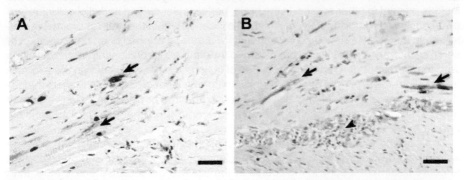

Fig. 1. (*A*) Biopsy from the proventriculus (pyloric area) of a healthy parrot. Note the presence of anti-CD117 brown-stained interstitial Cajal cells (ICC - *arrows*) interspersed through the smooth muscle cells of the proventriculus wall. (IHC by using anti CD117 as primary antibody; nuclear counterstain with Mayer's hematoxylin. Scale bar = 25 μm). (*B*) Biopsy from a pyloric area of the proventriculus of a PDD-affected parrot. Note the presence of anti-CD117 brown-stained interstitial Cajal cells (ICC - *arrows*) interspersed through the smooth muscle cells of the proventriculus, in which a lymphoplasmacytic inflammatory reaction is also present (*arrow-head*). (IHC by using anti CD117 as primary antibody; nuclear counterstain with Mayer's hematoxylin. Scale bar = 25 μm).

expands to the distal vagal ganglion or, from a mammalian perspective, the nodose ganglia near the thyroid gland. These ganglion cells are the cell bodies to afferent nerves (not efferents) of the parasympathetic nervous system. It is unknown if these ganglion cells are also affected by AG/PDD.

Several nerves branch from the nodose ganglion. One branch is the nerve to the carotid body, which receives sensory input. Some birds have nerve fibers that originate from the baroreceptors of the aortic and pulmonary roots to provide information on oxygenation. Those rootlets then send that information to the brainstem.

There are also fine filaments of nerve fibers that go to the glands of the neck that include the thyroid, parathyroid, and ultimobranchial bodies. The cranial cardiac nerve originates from the heart to join the vagus just distal to the distal vagal ganglion. The recurrent nerve anastomoses with the hypoglossal cervical nerve and distributes nerve fibers to the crop, esophagus, trachea, and syrinx, indicating a vast nerve supply from the vagus. This nerve continues as the pulmo esophageal nerve, sending fibers from the lungs that include information regarding CO_2 levels in the lung parenchyma. There are additional rami of pulmonary nerves from the vagus that supply the lungs as well. Additionally, 2 to 3 caudal cardiac nerves supply the heart.

From the study of Berhane and colleagues,[32] in a variety of parrots that were diagnosed with AG/PDD by histology, 79% had lymphoplasmatic infiltrates of the epicardial ganglia with additional infiltrates in the connective tissue between the myofibril bundles of the heart. In addition, myocardial necrosis with infiltration of mononuclear cells was observed histologically. The cardiac nerves supplying the heart were also affected, with the right more than the left. Lesions were more frequent and severe in the right side of the heart, which may reflect the higher density of nerves in this area. Arrhythmias and alterations in blood pressure also may be observed. Cardiac lesions can result in acute death in otherwise clinically normal birds. These histologic observations should be considered with cardiac workups. AG/PDD should be considered in the differential list of any bird exhibiting cardiac signs. Conversely, cardiac disease should be considered and evaluated in any parrot diagnosed with AG/PDD.

Central nervous system lesions commonly associated with AG involve the encephalon and/or cerebellum, and therefore suggest renaming this disease in addition to the lesions present in other organs. In the brain, perivascular cuffing and glial cell injury are often observed. Unfortunately, the anatomic location within the brain or brainstem was not described by Berhane and colleagues.[32] To date, there has been no evaluation of serial sections of the brain and brainstem to determine the relationship of clinical signs with the corresponding anatomic location of lesions observed. Based on the information to date, the changes of glial cell injury with myelin necrosis most likely is the underlying cause of seizures or ataxia observed in affected birds. Brain lesions also may affect areas involved in cognition, as some owners report that their bird suddenly is unable to recognize them or acts fearful when approached.

Cortical blindness, for example, has been presumed to occur as a consequence of lesions in the optic visual field areas of the telencephalon, which may be reversed with effective treatment if early in the course of the disease process. Blindness other than from optic nerve lesions is poorly described in birds, and the relationship of the areas in the brain that are affected by AG/PDD is not well known. Chorioretinitis has also been described.[33] Disruption of the Purkinje, glial, and granule cell layers of the cerebellum have been described in parrots with AG/PDD.[32] The Purkinje cells are inhibitory neurons that regulate and coordinate the normal movement of the body. Lesions of these cells and others in the cerebellar cortex produce disorders in fine movement and equilibrium, evidenced as ataxia, proprioceptive deficits, intention tremors, incoordination, dysarthria (vocalization abnormalities), and motor deficits. Old World psittacines often exhibit these central nervous system signs, although concurrent, nonclinical lesions in the GI tract are usually present (Orosz and Dahlhausen, personal communication).

Inflammation and myelin degeneration of the dorsal nerve roots, white matter, and associated ganglia have been identified at all levels of the spinal cord in AG/PDD-affected birds.[32] Mild to severe coalescing vacuolation and spongiosis of the white matter was observed in 5 of 9 birds examined. The gray matter was also affected. Thoracolumbar lesions were the most common and severe. The white matter consists of nerve tracts that send sensory and motor information to and from the brain and brainstem to the spinal cord. The dorsal root ganglia contain cell bodies of sensory neurons that bring information from the periphery to the spinal cord and then to the brain to understand the body wall and limbs in 3-dimensional space. Depending on the location of these lesions, this information can explain changes in the neurologic examination for posture and movement in affected birds, as well as sensory and motor ataxia. AG/PDD-associated peripheral neuritis also has been implicated as one cause of feather picking and self-mutilation in affected birds.[32]

A survey of pet birds with clinical signs of AG/PDD found 66% of birds exhibited central nervous system signs, 22% GI tract signs, 9% feather picking and mutilation, and 9% acute death.[34] For this reason, parrots with CNS signs and feather picking should include AG/PDD on the differential list.

PATHOLOGY

AG/PDD is a syndrome characterized by limited gross pathologic changes in affected birds. The macroscopic and microscopic lesions in birds with AG/PDD have been extensively studied.[35,36] Gross lesions include mild to severe emaciation; atrophy of the pectoral, proventricular, and ventricular muscles; proventricular dilatation; and duodenal distension.[32,37] Proventricular rupture and resulting peritonitis have been reported rarely. Occasionally, no gross lesions are observed.

Macroscopic lesions at necropsy are very few and, if the proventricular and intestinal dilatation are excluded, nonspecific. As reported by different researchers, 50% of birds presented for necropsy had pectoral muscle atrophy.[32] Occasionally, affected parrots may present a marked dilatation of the crop. This is most likely the result of lymphoplasmacytic perineural infiltration of the nerves to the crop. Additionally, there is often perivascular infiltration. For this reason, crop biopsies, sampled from the appropriate area surgically, may provide antemortem confirmation of the disease.

The presence of a dilated, thin-walled proventriculus with undigested food (**Fig. 2**) is considered a typical gross lesion associated with this disease. Radiographically, the proventriculus is considered dilated when the diameter of the organ is equal to or greater than the length of the femur (**Fig. 3**). Typically, the stomach develops a "J" shape, causing the ventriculus to be displaced to the right and ventrally (**Fig. 4**). In some parrots, the ventriculus is also thin-walled and distended, as well as the duodenal loop. Birds with only the neurologic form of this disease rarely show gross pathologic alterations, although Berhane and colleagues[32] described the presence of 0.2 to 1.0 mL of transparent fluid accumulated in the subarachnoid space in some birds. In the cardiac form of the disease, in which sudden death has occurred, the right ventricle of the heart may be dilated and thin-walled. As previously reported, lories (Loriidae) represent an exception in that proventricular/duodenal loop dilatation are generally absent. In these parrots, death occurs apparently for other causes, and necropsy does not show pathognomonic alterations of the gastrointestinal tract.[38]

AG/PDD is a disease in which histopathology represents the best way to evaluate the lesions and confirm a diagnosis. Microscopically, it is characterized by

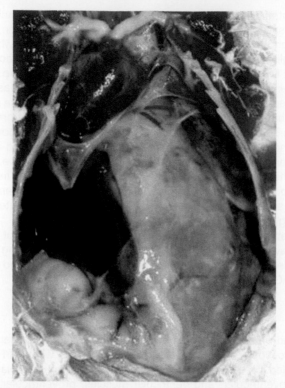

Fig. 2. Dilated, thin-walled proventriculus in an umbrella cockatoo (*Cacatua alba*).

nonsuppurative inflammation in peripheral, central, and autonomic nervous tissues.[10,32,39] Characteristic histologic lesions of AG/PDD involve lymphocytic, plasmacytic inflammatory infiltrates of nervous tissues, axonal swelling, myelin degeneration, and perivascular mononuclear cell infiltrates of blood vessels and connective tissue surrounding affected nerves (**Fig. 5**).[32]

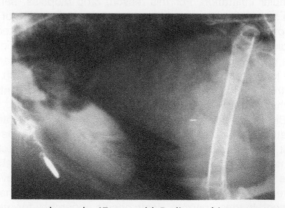

Fig. 3. *Poicephalus senegalus*, male, 17 years old. Radiographic appearance of a dilated proventriculus; note that the femur is use as a "scale bar" to evaluate the proventricular diameter. Generally, the proventriculus is considered dilated when the diameter of the organ is equal to or greater than the length of the femur.

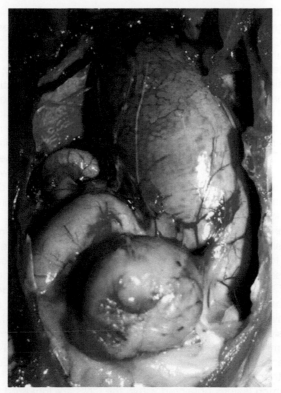

Fig. 4. Female, 12-year-old Illiger macaw (*Primolius maracana*) with gross lesions of AG/PDD. Note the characteristic "J" shape formed when the proventriculus is enlarged, displacing the ventriculus to the right and ventrally.

Lymphoplasmacytic infiltrates within myenteric ganglia and nerves of the proventriculus and ventriculus, and less frequently of the crop, esophagus, and duodenum, are the histologic hallmarks of AG/PDD and are considered pathognomonic for the disease by some investigators.[10,32,40] Similar infiltrates also may be present in the brain and spinal cord in the form of perivascular cuffing, and in peripheral nerves,[32,39]

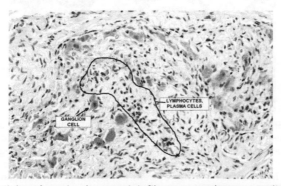

Fig. 5. Characteristic lymphocytic, plasmacytic infiltrate around nerve ganglia. (H&E stain. 40X.)

adrenal glands, myocardium, conductive tissue of the heart[17] and nerves or ganglia adjacent to various tissues, including adrenals, epicardium, and testes.[41] Nonsuppurative leiomyositis, polyserositis,[42] retinal degeneration, chorioretinitis[33,43] and perivascular dermatitis also have been described.[39,42]

Lesions are often present in ganglia of the GI tract (ganglioneuritis); central nervous system (encephalitis, myelitis); peripheral nerves, including the sciatic, brachial, and vagal nerves (neuritis); and retina (retinitis). Abnormalities may be observed at all levels of the spinal cord but are especially severe in the thoracolumbar portion. They include vacuolation and spongiosis of the white matter, axonal swelling with myelin degeneration, perivascular infiltrates in the gray and white matter and associated ganglia and dorsal nerve roots, and gliosis. Lesions also may be observed in the heart, which demonstrates focal to diffuse areas of myocardial necrosis associated with infiltration of mononuclear cells. The intracardiac nerve plexus of the right side of the heart is often more severely affected.[17] Lymphocytes may be scattered diffusely throughout the adrenal medulla or localized in clusters adjacent to cortical tissue.

The most important and consistent histopathological lesions present are in the CNS and PNS. Generally, AG/PDD-associated neural lesions are characterized by degeneration and mild to moderate neuronal spongiosis, apoptosis and neuronal necrosis, neuronophagia, satellitosis, and gliosis. Anecdotally, there is a tendency to exclude the presence of lesions at the axonal level, and, in particular, demyelination as disease-related lesions. Recently, de Araujo and colleagues,[44] in an ABV review, argued that demyelinating lesions are not part of the AG/PDD pathology, whereas demyelinating lesions have been repeatedly described by various investigators.[32,45,46] Regarding the immune phenotypization of the mononuclear cell infiltrates, it is possible to observe strong macrophagic activity around myelin fibers with macrophages laden with myelin residue in the cytoplasm (Figs. 6 and 7).[45,46]

The most common lesions observed within the CNS are localized in the cerebrum and are characterized by a nonsuppurative encephalitis with associated perivascular cuffing. Cerebellar lesions are characterized by focal gliosis, some perivascular cuffing, and Purkinje cell necrosis or interruptions. Perivascular cuffing, frequently associated with neuronal pathology in the brain, is constituted primarily of lymphocytes

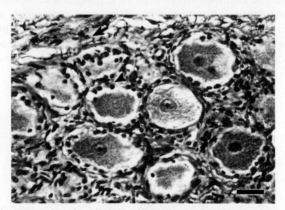

Fig. 6. Adrenal gland ganglia of a AG/PDD-affected parrot, stained with Luxol fast blue and Cresyl violet. The section shows a sleeve of demyelination and inflammation represented by mononuclear cell accumulation (particularly lymphocytes) inside the ganglion and around neurons (*chevron*). Reduced staining by Luxol fast blue indicates a decreased presence of myelin. Myelin fragmentation is also evident (*arrow*). *Arrowhead* head indicates myelin fragmentation. (Scale bar = 25 μm).

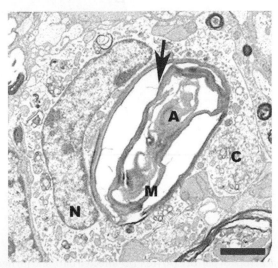

Fig. 7. Ultrastructural examination of a peripheral nerve with a severe damage induced by macrophage phagocytosis of a myelinated axon in an AG/PDD-affected parrot. Note the swollen axon with myelin degeneration during phagocytosis (*arrow*). A, axon; C, macrophage cytoplasm; M, myelin; N, macrophage nucleus. (Scale bar = 2 μm.)

and macrophages, typically CD3/CD8-positive and CD68/Lysozyme/AF488-positive cells.[45–47] These perivascular mononuclear cell aggregates are also observed near the Purkinje cell layer of the cerebellum. Immunohistochemical studies performed using anti-ABV N-protein antibody have shown scattered antigen-positive glia in the cerebrum, with many of these cells exhibiting cytoplasmic vacuolization. Antigen-positive cells in the cerebellum are generally found in highest density in the Purkinje cell layer. Weak axonal staining is observed when staining the molecular layer.

Lesions associated with other organs are well characterized, particularly in the GI tract. Pesaro and colleagues[47] described alterations occurring in the crop of parrots affected by AG/PDD. In particular, this present study reports, for the first time, a decrease in the number of proliferating cellular nuclear antigen (PCNA)-positive cells in the basal layer of the crop epithelium (**Fig. 8**), associated with a reduction in thickness of superficial prekeratinized layer in affected parrots (**Fig. 9**). PCNA was originally described as an antigen that is expressed in the nuclei of cells during the DNA synthesis phase of the cell cycle.[48] PCNA is a DNA clamp that acts as a processivity factor, enhancing DNA polymerase δ enzyme in eukaryotic cells' ability to catalyze consecutive reactions without releasing its substrate. It is essential for replication, acting as a scaffold to recruit proteins involved in DNA replication, DNA repair, chromatin remodeling, and epigenetics.[49] Lymphomononuclear cell, perigangliar infiltrate, typical of AG/PDD was also identified in these tissues.

A decrease of PCNA expression in the basal layer of crop's epithelium indicates a decrease in the cellular turnover rate. In association with the previously mentioned findings, this may represent a nonspecific, early disease sign, related to the dystrophic status of the crop wall caused by the nonsuppurative ganglioneuritis. The progressive and severe thinning and atrophy of the crop wall, associated with organ dilatation and dyskinesia, could be the consequence of these primary histologic alterations. Similar changes are observed in human skin during neuropathies.[50] In individuals with

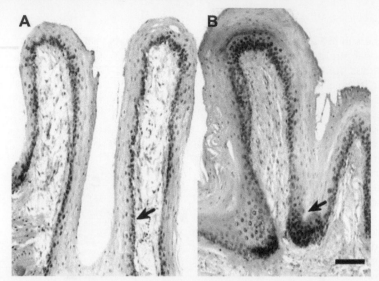

Fig. 8. Biopsies from 2 crops of parrots. (*A*) AG/PDD-affected bird, and (*B*) healthy parrot. Note a strong reduction of cells that show PCNA expression at the nuclear level (*arrow in A*) into the basal layer of the crop's epithelium of a parrot with AG/PDD, versus normal expression (*arrow in B*) in the healthy control. This indicates decreased cellular turnover in the crop epithelium of AG/PDD-affected parrots. (IHC performed using anti PCNA, clone Ki67, as primary antibody; nuclear counterstain with Mayer's hematoxylin. Scale bar = 400 μm.)

diabetic neuropathy and ulceration, a reduced epidermal thickness was demonstrated at the pulp of the big toe as the result of increased subepidermal edema and loss of intradermal small nervous fibers. Small fiber neuropathy results from selective impairment of small myelinated A-delta and unmyelinated C fibers. The density of small

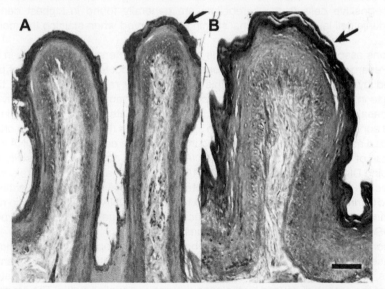

Fig. 9. Biopsies from 2 crops of parrots. (*A*) AG/PDD-affected bird, and (*B*) healthy parrot. Note a reduction in thickness of superficial prekeratinized layer in the affected parrot (*left arrow*), with respect to a healthy bird (*right arrow*). (HC performed using a Dane and Herman's tetra chromic stain. Scale bar = 400 μm.)

nerve fibers in the epidermis is severely reduced and the skin over the affected area may appear atrophic, dry, shiny, and discolored.[51]

Numerous publications have documented a high percentage of CD3+ cells in the periganglial infiltrate with a large presence of CD8+ T cells and macrophages in affected and symptomatic birds (**Fig. 10**). As in the proventriculus, gizzard, and intestine, the correlation between immunophenotypic findings and morphologic data indicate microscopic changes characterized by a nonsuppurative ganglioneuritis with gliosis, cuffing, focal areas of demyelination, and ganglial swelling.[3,32,35,39]

The immunohistochemical characterization of inflammatory cell populations in addition to histologic patterns observed in altered crop tissue is suggestive of viral-induced damage, in association with an immune-mediated mechanism of disease. However, the histologic pattern does not exclude the implication of ABV or other biological agents still not recognized, in initiating the process of priming lymphocytes against self-antigens, such as myelin components and/or gangliosides (GSLs).[16,52–54] Severity of crop dystrophy and inflammatory perineural infiltration are strictly related to the clinical signs of the disease and to the ABV infective condition.[47] In asymptomatic parrots that show initial AG/PDD-related lesions at crop biopsy, the perineural/perivascular infiltrates are generally characterized by a low percentage of CD3+ lymphocytes, with a variable percentage of plasma cells and macrophages. Only occasional CD8+ cells (granzyme-positive cytotoxic T lymphocytes) and macrophages are observed mixed with scattered CD3+ T cells. Conversely, in the symptomatic birds, infiltrates are characterized by a large percentage of CD8+ lymphocytes and macrophages (see **Fig. 10**). It is of interest to note that the average number of PCNA-positive cells counted in affected crop samples in this study was 75.8 cells per ×40 high-power field (HPF). The value obtained in samples belonging to asymptomatic, unaffected parrots (186.6 PCNA-positive cells per ×40 HPF) is more than double the value of the cell population count in the affected parrots. Notably, in cells of the basal layer, PCNA count varied independently to the degree of the pathology and the severity of the lymphoid infiltrate

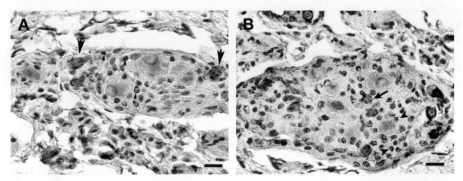

Fig. 10. (*A*) Immunophenotype of mononuclear cells that infiltrate a proventricular ganglion of a parrot affected by early stage of AG/PDD; note the presence of CD8+/granzyme+ lymphocytes (stained in blue) (*little arrows*) interspersed inside the ganglion and between neurons, in association with macrophages (stained in brown) (*big arrows*) and CD3+ lymphocytes (unstained). (*B*) Immunophenotype of mononuclear cells that infiltrate a proventricular ganglion of a parrot with clinical AG/PDD of one year's duration. Note the appearance of CD4+ lymphocytes (stained in red with blue; chevrons), interspersed with CD8+/granzyme+ lymphocytes (stained in blue), admixed with macrophages (stained in brown, *arrow*) inside the ganglion and between damaged neurons. (IHC performed using anti granzyme, anti F40/80, and anti CD4 as primary antibodies; nuclear counterstain with Mayer's hematoxylin. Scale bar = 40 μm).

in the 2 groups. Similarly, specimens stained with a particular stain for keratinized epithelium show a different thickness in prekeratinized epithelial layer of the crop between groups, with an evident thinness of this stratum in affected birds (see **Fig. 9**).

As previously mentioned, pathologic lesions of AG/PDD are found within the CNS, including the cerebellum. Cerebellar lesions are dominated by Purkinje cell necrosis, neuronophagia, myelin degeneration, gliosis, and axonal swelling that sometimes accompany the inflammatory neural lesions.[32] The frequency and extent of inflammation in various organs and in the different parts of the brain and spinal cord have been described by several investigators.[4,29,32,35,39] These vary greatly, are not consistent among cases, and often do not reflect the type or severity of clinical signs or observed gross lesions.[32] Whether there is a relationship between lesions and species of bird affected or stage of the disease is not known.[32,41] Immunohistochemical studies reveal the expression of ABV N-protein in the cerebrum, with antigen staining most intense within nuclei, and cytoplasm of some vacuolated neurons and in many glial cells. Within the cerebellum, ABV N-protein is instead found most consistently within cells of the Purkinje cell layer. Although no Purkinje cells contain viral antigen, the presence of significant interruptions in the Purkinje cell layer and increase in apoptosis suggests that they are adversely affected by this virus. The cells adjacent to the Purkinje cells are commonly observed to be antigen-positive and many show evidence of degeneration. The precise nature of the target cells in the cerebellum is unclear, but we speculate that immune-mediated processes are involved in the Purkinje cell layer damage and this Purkinje cell loss may be secondary to the immune-mediated destruction.

PATHOGENESIS
Avian Bornavirus

An infectious etiology for AG/PDD has long been suspected based on its apparent spread through aviary collections. Transmission electron microscopy studies in the 1990s provided the first evidence of a viral etiology demonstrating inclusion bodies and enveloped viruslike particles in the myenteric plexus, celiac ganglia, and fresh feces from affected birds.[55] Attempts to isolate an infectious agent were unsuccessful at that time.

In 2008, 2 independent research groups identified a novel virus in tissues from AG/PDD-affected birds and named it avian *bornavirus* (ABV).[52,53] It was proposed as the causative agent of AG/PDD. Subsequent studies have confirmed the association between ABV infection and AG/PDD.[16,37,54–59] Disease development was reproduced by parenteral inoculation of psittacine birds, such as cockatiels (*Nymphicus hollandicus*) or Patagonian conures (*Cyanoliseus patagonus*), with genotypes ABV-2 and ABV-4. However, ABV has also been found in healthy birds that may remain apparently disease-free for years.[16,54,56,57]

Bornaviruses are enveloped, nonsegmented single-stranded negative-sense RNA viruses. They are members of the family Bornaviridae in the order Mononegavirales. Other families within the order include the Filoviridae (West Nile virus), Rhabdoviridae (rabies virus), and the Paramyxoviridae. To date, 15 genetically diverse ABVs, which comprise 6 distinct viral species, have been identified. The recent reclassification of ABVs is psittaciform bornavirus 1 (which includes parrot bornavirus [PaBV] 1, 2, 3, 4, 7), passeriform bornavirus 1 (CnBV-1, 2, 3, canary) and (MuBV-1, munia finch), waterbird bornavirus 1 (ABBV-1, aquatic bird bornavirus 1), passeriform bornavirus 2 (EsBV-1,estrildid finch bornavirus 1), and tentative, unclassified bornaviruses of ABV-MALL, parrot bornavirus 5 PaBV-5, parrot bornavirus 6 PaBV-6, and parrot bornavirus 8 PaBV-8.[34,59,60] PaBV-2 and PaBV-4 are the predominate genotypes infecting birds. Analysis of N gene sequences from PaBV-4 shows that PaBV-4 is further separated into 5 distinct clusters, whereas PaBV-2 does not clearly separate into distinct groups. The classification of PaBV-5 and PaBV-6 is tentative and remains unclassified at the species level.

The genetic variability of ABV is much greater than that observed in borna disease virus. There is a 91% to 100% shared nucleotide identity within a genotype and only 68% to 85% between genotypes. Different genotypes seem to cause different disease in different species and individuals but the relationship among genotype, species of bird, and observed clinical disease is obscure at this time. One induced infection study in cockatiels demonstrated that more birds displayed clinical signs and disease progression was more severe in birds infected with PaBV-2 compared with PaBV-4.[61] Clinically, different courses of disease were also observed. PaBV-2 infection mainly affected the gastrointestinal tract, whereas more neurologic signs were noted with PaBV-4 infection. Infection with one genotype does not appear to be protective against another. Simultaneous infection with 2 genotypes can occur and may result in severely worse clinical disease.

ABV is widely distributed in the body of infected birds.[62] It reproduces in a noncytopathic manner in the host nucleus and persists due to mechanisms that evade the host immune system.[63] As a result, ABV infections are considered chronic and lifelong. It is therefore unlikely that antiviral or vaccine therapy will effectively eliminate the viral infected state.

Infection Rate

ABV is widely distributed in both captive and wild avian populations. Approximately 15% to 40% of normal healthy birds are positive for the presence of ABV. Lierz[64] detected ABV RNA in 27 (45.8%) of 59 healthy appearing pet birds. Thirty-five (45%) of 77 healthy birds from an aviary with a past history of AG/PDD were found positive for ABV-specific serum antibodies.[65] A survey of laboratory samples submitted for other testing revealed approximately 34% (271/791) avian samples tested positive from across the United States.[66]

Almost all collections of psittacine birds will contain individuals infected with ABV. A large-scale survey revealed that ABV infection is widespread among captive psittacines in Europe, with 23% of 1442 birds considered infected.[56] Similarly, a high infection rate was observed in captive canaries in Germany and in certain populations of wild waterfowl in North America.[67,68]

Although a significant percentage of the avian population is infected with ABV, the frequency of clinical borna viral disease is much lower. Most ABV-positive birds do not exhibit clinical disease. When it does occur, disease presents on a continuum of intensity with many birds exhibiting only mild disease. The clinically "wasted" bird represents the more severe form of untreated, chronic disease.

Transmission

The epidemiology of ABV is currently not well understood. The virus is shed in the urine and feces of infected birds.[60,62,69] The urofecal-oral route is therefore assumed to be important for the horizontal transmission of the virus. However, support of this premise by scientific study is ambiguous. Kistler and colleagues[70] documented the rapid spread of ABV infection among juvenile birds in a psittacine nursery. The outbreak resulted in the acute disease and death of 13 unweaned chicks of various species. Another report by Piepenbring and colleagues[57] documented the successful transmission of ABV to one cockatiel placed in contact with a group of cockatiels experimentally infected with PaBV-4. Most other studies indicate that horizontal transmission of ABV by direct contact is inefficient in immunocompetent, fully fledged birds.[69] Cockatiels were infected with PaBV-4 by oral and intranasal application. Clinical signs of disease were not observed in any of the birds during the 174-day observation period. At the end of the study, patho-histological and immunohistochemical examination revealed neither lesions typical for AG/PDD nor ABV-specific antigen in any of the birds.[71] These observations suggest that ABV transmission may be much more efficient in unweaned nestlings with immaturely developed immune systems compared with older individuals. The proposed fecal-oral transmission mode as the natural route of infection in immunocompetent adult or subadult cockatiels is not supported in this study. It should be noted that it is commonly observed that birds exposed to naturally or experimentally infected cagemates remain virus-free for extended periods.[69,72] Phylogenetic analysis of PaBV-2, PaBV-4, and ABBV-1 sequences obtained in a study of captive and free-ranging birds and reported GenBank sequences found identical or genetically closely related ABV sequences in parallel in various species. The authors conclude that interspecies spread is a frequent occurrence relative to the overall transmission of ABV and supports the horizontal mode of viral transmission.[73]

Experimental studies have shown that ABV infections can be induced experimentally when the virus is injected intramuscularly, intravenously, and/or intracranially in birds. Gancz and colleagues[37] were the first to demonstrate that AG/PDD could be transmitted to healthy birds by the use of infected brain tissue. They inoculated cockatiels by multiple routes with a brain homogenate from either an PaBV-4–positive bird or from an AG/PDD-/ABV-control bird. The birds inoculated with healthy control bird homogenate remained healthy, whereas all 3 birds inoculated with brain homogenate from ABV-infected birds developed both gross and microscopic lesions typical of AG/PDD.[37] Gray and colleagues[58] isolated ABV in cultured duck embryo fibroblasts. After 6 passages, these infected cells were injected intramuscularly into 2 Patagonian conures. Clinical signs of AG/PDD developed within 66 days postinfection in both challenged birds. The presence of typical AG/PDD lesions was demonstrated on necropsy and histopathology. Reverse-transcriptase polymerase chain reaction (RT-PCR) documented the presence of the inoculated ABV in the brains of the challenged birds.[58] Piepenbring and colleagues[57] inoculated 18 cockatiels by both the intracerebral and intravenous routes with an isolate of PaBV-4 cultured for 6 passages in a quail cell line (CEC-32). All challenged birds became persistently infected, but the clinical disease patterns that developed varied among individuals. Five birds developed clinical signs of AG/PDD, whereas on necropsy 7 of the 18 had a dilated proventriculus. All infected birds did, however, show mononuclear cell infiltrates characteristic of AG/PDD in a wide range of organs.[57]

Other routes of viral transmission cannot be excluded. Spread via the respiratory tract and vertically through the egg have been discussed. Strong suggestive evidence for vertical transmission of ABV from the hen to the egg has been reported in psittacines and canaries. Several studies found eggs from infected hens to be ABV-positive by PCR assays.[69,74–76] Final proof of vertical transmission provided by the detection of productive infection in embryos or chicks reared under isolated conditions is lacking at this time.

Incubation Period

The incubation period of AG/PDD is unknown. Clinical observations suggest that this could be as short as several weeks to as long as many years.[8,77] In general, transmission is believed to require long-term, close contact among birds. Unlike other RNA viruses that are more stable (West Nile Virus), endonuclease enzymes in the environment tend to rapidly degrade the ABV. Soap and dilute bleach appear to be effective in disinfecting enclosures and items that come in contact with ABV-positive individuals. The sensitivity of ABV to desiccation suggests that virus could lose viability soon after being shed into the environment.[78]

Role of Avian Bornavirus in Pathogenesis of Avian Ganglioneuritis/ Proventricular Dilatation Disease

Despite numerous studies published on AG/PDD and its association with ABV, the pathogenesis of this disease remains unclear. Although the first reports of ABV in AG/PDD-affected parrots suggested that ABV was a plausible cause of AG/PDD, full proof of a causal relationship using Koch's postulates required isolation of the agent trom infected birds, its propagation in culture and manifestation of the disease after reintroduction of the isolate into a susceptible host. These postulates were fulfilled when cockatiels (*N hollandicus*) and Patagonian conures (*Cyanoliseus patagonus*) were inoculated with cultured ABV genotype 4 via intramuscular (IM), intracerebral, and intravenous (IV) routes and disease resulted.[57,58,79,80] AG/PDD has also been reproduced in cockatiels inoculated with brain homogenate containing ABV genotype 4 via combined IM, intraocular, intranasal, and oral routes[37] and with cultured ABV genotype 2 via combined oral and IM, IV, and intracerebral routes.[79,81] The results of these experiments support a causal relationship between ABV and AG/ PDD in psittacine birds.

Asymptomatic Infection with Avian Bornavirus

In spite of infection studies with ABV that have satisfied Koch's postulates, and the opinion of some researchers that ABV is the sole cause of AG/PDD,[82] the relationship of ABV in the pathogenesis of this disease is controversial. In fact, more recently, successful inoculation of canaries with cultured ABV-C2 via IM, subcutaneous, oral, and oculo-nasal routes have been documented: interestingly, shedding of virus, seroconversion, and re-isolation of ABV-C2 from the brains of inoculated birds occurred but no signs of clinical disease or macroscopic lesions attributable to ABV infection were observed in any of the inoculated birds. Histopathological changes consistent with AG/PDD were minimal.[69] Additionally, during a trial in specific pathogen-free Mallard ducklings (*Anas platyrhynchos*) inoculated with cultured psittacine ABV genotype 4, the investigators documented viral shed in the feces and seroconversion in infected birds within 3 weeks. Inoculation did not result in disease based on a lack of clinical signs and histopathological lesions on necropsy, 8 months after inoculation.[83] Similarly, rats and mice challenged with ABV-4 did not develop clinical signs or lesions.[84]

Asymptomatic ABV infection has been identified in both experimentally and naturally infected birds and likely plays an important role in the epidemiology of AG/ PDD.[35,37,70,72,79] Many apparently healthy psittacines carry ABV for prolonged periods. In a recent study, ABV was detected in 40% (12/30) of sampled captive canary flocks in Germany, with most of these birds healthy and exhibiting no apparent clinical disease.[67] The exact factors that trigger the development of lesions or clinical signs are unknown. Experimentally, Borna disease development varies with host species, age, and immune system function.[69] Age at infection may determine the rate of progression of disease in ABV-infected birds. Younger birds appear to have a more rapid course of disease progression than older birds.[70] Vertical transmission of borna disease virus (BDV) has been demonstrated in mammals and is believed to occur with ABV in birds.[67,74,75,85] This transmission route may also play an important role in the outcome of infection. It is also possible that the ABV genotype affects the form of clinical disease. Although a direct relationship between genotype and virulence has not been formally demonstrated,[37,80] a recent study suggests that there may be differences in pathogenicity among ABV isolates with cockatiels infected with ABV-2 showing earlier and more severe clinical symptoms compared with birds infected with ABV-4.[79]

Proposed Autoimmune Mechanisms for Avian Ganglioneuritis/ Proventricular Dilatation Disease

The mechanisms involved in the development of CNS lesions are readily understood only in those pathologic conditions in which there is evidence that a virus destroys its target cell as a direct cytopathic consequence of viral replication. The lesions and symptoms seen with BDV of mammals in experimentally infected rodents are the result of neural invasion by CD8 T lymphocytes and subsequent cytotoxicity, rather than virus-inflicted cellular damage.[86–90] Thus, it is generally believed that bornavirus infection–related lesions are in large part immunologically mediated.[90–93] The mechanism through which ABV causes the lesions and clinical syndrome of AG/PDD remains unclear; however, a similar immune-mediated pathogenesis is likely.[37] Several recent communications have suggested that an autoimmune mechanism (production of autoreactive anti-GSL antibodies, complement activation, and a cell-mediated immune-response activation), similar to that observed in Guillain-Barré syndrome (GBS) in humans, is involved in the pathogenesis of AG/PDD.[46,94–97] The disease process of AG/PDD appears to involve inflammation of the nerve ganglia, which exposes normally sequestered GSL proteins to the host immune system. Rossi and colleagues[45–47,94,95] have shown that the release of G 50 proteins from nerve ganglia produce pathologic lesions similar to those noted in the autoimmune neuropathy of GBS. Disease is suggested to occur when the host immune response is directed to these exposed proteins causing corresponding neurologic dysfunction. The detection of anti-GSL antibodies in the sera of AG/PDD-affected birds and the successful reproduction of AG/PDD via inoculation of purified GSLs into healthy cockatiels support this theory.[95]

Recently, in an attempt to demonstrate the absence of any correlation between the development of anti-GSL antibodies in sera of AG/PDD-affected parrots and pathogenesis of AG/PDD lesions, de Araujo and colleagues[44] described an experimental inoculation of chickens and Quaker parrots (*Myiopsitta monachus*) with GSLs purified from parrot CNS. The inoculation of these antigens, admixed in Freund's complete adjuvant, was done as described previously by Rossi and colleagues.[95,96]

Although the authors conclude that there was no correlation between the development of clinical or pathologic signs related to the inoculation,[44] the development of CNS and PNS mononuclear cell infiltrates in inoculated birds were observed. The mild perivascular and perineural lymphocytic infiltrate in the proventriculus of inoculated chickens, as well as minimal to mild, focal, lymphocytic aggregates found in the cerebrum are arbitrarily considered by the authors to be physiologic lymphoid aggregates, occasionally observed in the gastrointestinal tract or in CNS of avian species.[98] Similarly, a Quaker parrot developed mild, multifocal, lymphoplasmacytic encephalitis in the optic tectum, and mild, multifocal lymphoplasmacytic and histiocytic myelitis in the thoracic and lumbar segments after GSL inoculation. Any relationship between the development of these lesions and the GSL inoculation was discounted in this study.

The conclusions of de Araujo and colleagues[44] are that most experimental studies involving PaBV inoculation in psittacine birds were able to induce the first clinical signs of AG/PDD, including depression, regurgitation, and undigested seeds in the feces, between 21 and 66 days after inoculation.[10,37,44,58] Bibliographic citations document only experiments in which the infection with ABV supported the development of AG/PDD. There are many other studies mentioned earlier that clearly show that no clinical signs or histologic lesions have occurred in birds after inoculation of ABV.[63,84] In general, ABV infection studies have relied on the injection of birds with large amounts of virus, not typical of exposures that may occur naturally. In addition, natural infections of ABV causing clinical AG/PDD are rare in the cockatiel, the species most commonly used in these trials.[69]

The major criticisms observed in the study by de Araujo and colleagues[44] are that it has not taken into account (1) the species of parrots that were used for GSL inoculation; (2) the age of parrots at the time of inoculation; (3) the arbitrary interpretation as *"physiologic lymphoid aggregates"* of the lesions observed in CNS and PNS of birds experimentally inoculated with GSLs; and (4) the absence of any immune-characterization of the lymphoid cells constituting these *"para-physiological"* infiltrates. As previously reported, the appearance of clinical symptoms and the development of histopathological lesions, even after infection with PaBV, is strictly dependent on host species, age, and immune function.[52,69,79]

Rossi and colleagues[95] evidenced different results in young cockatiels inoculated with purified GSLs or with GSLs pool extracted from CNS of ABV-uninfected parrots. Inoculated cockatiels showed a greater prevalence of characteristic clinical signs of AG/PDD and the development of typical histologic lesions. A constant element that unites the studies by de Araujo and colleagues[44] and Rossi and colleagues[95] is the development of a high anti-GSL antibody titer after GSL inoculation. However, it is unclear how significant these antibodies are, whether they develop secondary to tissue damage, and how they contribute to the disease process. Although AG/PDD is very unlikely to be an autoimmune disease per se, transient autoimmune responses occur in some AG/PDD cases and may contribute to the complex pathogenesis of this disease.[99]

The Complement System and Its Proposed Role in Pathogenesis of Lesions

The complement system, one of the most sophisticated innate immune systems of mammals and birds, was studied intensively from an evolutionary viewpoint.[100,101] Mammals, Aves, Amphibia, and Teleostei have a full set of complement genes. Brain cells, particularly microglia, are able to synthesize complement (C) components in response to experimental lesions.[102] Because C components not only participate in cytotoxic mechanisms and phagocytosis but also function as chemical mediators of inflammation (eg, C3a and C5a), it is likely that locally synthesized C components and C regulators may be central to the amplification and persistence of inflammatory processes in the CNS.[103–105] According to the results obtained from a large number of parrots with naturally occurring AG/PDD, anti-GSL antibodies are able to reach damaged CNS and PNS cells and activate the complement (C') cascade.[26] Rossi and colleagues[46] (2011) demonstrated strong C3 and C1q expression in tissues of parrots with lymphoplasmacytic ganglioneuritis, in areas of the CNS. This underscores the important role of complement activation in the pathogenesis of lesions related to the ABV infection. Immunohistological analysis of coronal sections of the brain belonging to ABV-infected parrots with central neurologic clinical signs ("neurologic forms") revealed the accumulation of C1q-positive cells throughout the gray and white matter. The highest accumulation of C3 and C1q-positive cells was seen in the hippocampal region and in the cortex. In the hippocampus, diffuse extracellular C1q immunostaining was also detected. Additional areas with a high density of C1q immunostaining included the hypothalamus, juxtaventricular regions, and the basal cortex.

Normally, similar brain sections from uninfected parrots reveal only very low C' fraction expression. The enhanced expression of C' fractions from ABV-infected

CNS and PNS tissues coincides with the development of neurologic disease. The localization of increased Clq expression within those brain regions most afflicted with lesions (eg, hippocampus, basolateral cortex) suggests that locally produced complement might play a critical role in the initiation and amplification of inflammatory processes in the brain. Although ABV is noncytopathic, it can induce inflammation and a selective loss of glial cells and neurons. This cell loss appears secondary to T-cell cytotoxicity, which suggests that the local expression of C' in the CNS is unlikely to be directly induced by the virus. The presence of a clear C' expression (mostly C3) in strict association with T cells confirms that T-cell activity may be a stimulus. The collagenlike Clq molecule is the recognition subunit of the first component (Cl) of the classical complement pathway.[105] Because expression of other components, such as C3, is also increased inside central and peripheral areas of ABV-related lesions, it is possible that the classic or alternative complement pathways may actually become involved. There is suggestive evidence that C' activation is associated with a variety of human neurodegenerative diseases, such as Alzheimer disease,[106,107] as well as Parkinson disease, Huntington disease, and amyotrophic lateral sclerosis.[107] Similar observations were described in rats experimentally infected by borna disease virus. In this model, the potential role of C' components in the development of neurodegenerative disease was described.[105] With respect to our observations in parrots' central and peripheral nervous systems, brain expression levels of C3 were at least 10 times lower than those of Clq. From this evidence, the investigators concluded that the role of Clq in CNS inflammation may involve mechanisms other than a full complement cascade. The Clq is thought to play an important role in the adhesion of macrophages to the extracellular matrix, in cell-to-cell interactions between macrophages and other cell types (eg, fibroblasts), and therefore in processes involved in inflammation and tissue destruction.[108] Second, Clq can interact with a variety of cells in a receptor-mediated fashion to stimulate particular cell functions. For example, binding of Clq to monocytes results in the enhancement of monocyte phagocytic activity and cell surface–bound Clq can stimulate an oxidative burst in human neutrophils.[109,110] C3 accumulation was also evidenced, particularly in peripheral areas of nonsuppurative ganglionitis (**Fig. 11**).

Many studies of BDV pathogenesis have been performed in mammals, particularly in horses, ruminants, mice, rats, and humans. In these species, the mechanism of neuronal damage induced by virus infection is well known; BDV elicits limited pathology in the peripheral or central nervous system per se, but the immune response that fights the virus can cause severe CNS damage. Chronic CNS infection might also lead to secondary autoreactive T-cell responses that accelerate CNS damage. In most infectious disease models, CD8+ and CD4+ T cells are essential for virus control, but also significantly contribute to tissue destruction, whereas B cells appear to primarily control the virus during subacute or chronic CNS infection.

In a high percentage of parrots examined for gross and/or histologic lesions referable to parrot ganglioneuritis, the increased concentration of complement fraction expressions was associated with a strong infiltrate of lymphocytes and macrophages (**Fig. 12**). However, the outcome of ABV infection is variable depending on factors such as the host age, host genetic factors, and neurovirulence of the isolate (PaBV 1, 2, 3, 4, and so forth). Studies in rats and mice indicate that immunopathology in classic disease is mediated chiefly by N protein–specific CD8+ T cells. Interestingly, acute disease can recede despite persistence of replicating virus. This apparent tolerance is associated with a shift from a Th1-weighted to Th2-weighted immune response but the basis for this shift is unexplained. Transgenic mice expressing

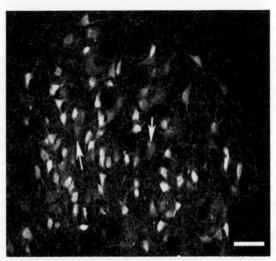

Fig. 11. Biopsy sample from the crop of an AG/PDD-affected parrot: note the strong expression of C3 fraction of the complement system, stained with an anti-C3 rhodamine conjugated specific antibody, between gangliar neurons. Cellular nuclei are counterstained with ab138903 Nuclear yellow (Hoechst 769121 - *arrows*). (IF performed using anti-C3 rhodamine conjugated specific antibody, ab138903 Nuclear yellow nuclear counterstain. Scale bar = 100 μm).

BDV N protein in either neurons or astrocytes are resistant to disease, presumably because of immunologic tolerance.[111]

Lesion Characterization in Parrots and Ganglioside Sensitization of the Host

In one of the authors' experience (Rossi) with AG/PDD-affected parrots with or without evidence of ABV infection, peripheral lesions are characterized by the early activation of CD8+ T (perforin/granzyme+) cells. The presence of CD8+ T cells parallels the onset of neurologic dysfunction, and directly targets ganglia and neurons, associated with vigorous CD4+ T-cell responses that recruit macrophages (see **Fig. 10**). This leads to the release of inflammatory mediators and toxic molecules, causing binding

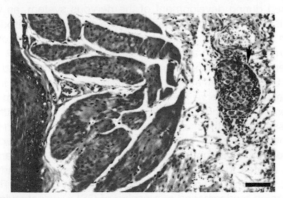

Fig. 12. Histologic lesions from the crop of a parrot with AG/PDD. There is an increased concentration of complement fraction expression associated with large numbers of lymphocytes and macrophages infiltrating a ganglion (*arrow*). (H&E stain. Scale bar = 500 μm).

of antibodies to neuronal surface antigens. This results in complement activation or antibody-mediated phagocytosis of axons. In birds with clinical AG/PDD, we demonstrated immunocomplex deposition around affected nerve ganglia associated with high positive expression of complement fractions by immunofluorescence.[46]

Although sequential events of CNS and PNS pathogenesis and immunophenotype characterization of inflammatory cells have been reported primarily in mouse and rat models, our immunohistochemical data provide insight into the mechanisms responsible for ABV damage in parrots. They provide evidence that CD8+/granzyme+ cells are responsible for the early events of neuronal damage and are predisposed to the delivery of neuronal components that sensitize the parrots. Immunocharacterization of the mononuclear cells that are constantly associated with CNS and PNS lesions in parrots with clinical AG/PDD indicate that the immunopathology is similar to BDV and is mediated by CD8+ T cells with help from CD4+ T-cell subsets. These CD8+ T cells demonstrate active cytolytic activity and are granzyme positive against target cells infected with ABV or those expressing BDV antigens.[46] Macrophages have an essential role in the development of nerve lesions in BDV and AG/PDD. They produce neuronophagia and axonal demyelination, inducing delivery of some cellular components, such as neural GSLs.[112–116] In birds, the lesions caused by ABV consist of a lymphoplasmacytic infiltrate, constituted by CD8+, CD4+, and CD68/Lysozyme/AF488-positive macrophages, in either the CNS or PNS (Rossi and colleagues,[95] 2008; Kistler and colleagues,[52] 2008; Staeheli, Rinder & Kaspers,[116] 2010). Although demyelination is not a predominant feature of AG/PDD, it is observed and documented by transmission electron microscopy (see **Fig. 7**). Indirect mechanisms, such as loss of protective myelin by macrophages, mitochondrial dysfunction, or release of glutamate or nitric oxide, may also contribute to axonal damage. Although these mechanisms could be relevant, the molecular events that underlie the axonal damage in AG/PDD are represented by GSL sensitization of the host.

GSLs are major components of neuronal membranes, where they contribute up to 10% to 12% of the total lipid content and participate in crucial processes of the nervous system.[117] They are integral components of the nerve plasma membrane, distinguishing surface markers that can serve as specific determinants in cellular recognition and modulation of cell signal transduction events. More than 60 GSLs are known, which vary among nervous system structures and among different species. Recently, GSLs have been found to be highly important molecules in immunology. Their regulatory roles are suggested by the dramatic change in the pattern of GSLs expressed during development of the nervous system, as well as by their region-specific distribution.[118] The variation of these molecules throughout development and life can account for the variable distribution and severity of lesions in AG/PDD-affected parrots of varying age and species.

The brain content of GSLs changes throughout life, during aging and in neurodegenerative diseases. One important aspect of GSL-mediated cell-to-cell interaction is the organization of myelinated nerve fibers. The interaction between myelin sheet and axon is critical for axonal trophic support. Neuronal GSLs, in particular GM1, GD1a, and GT1b, are essential for the maintenance of myelinated axons in the central and peripheral nervous system. GM1, which is enriched in paranodal structures, is critical for the cytoarchitecture of paranodal regions.[119] Interestingly, disorganization of paranodal structures, related to a GM1 loss, have been observed in early lesions in the brains of patients with multiple sclerosis (MS) before demyelination. These abnormalities are accompanied by decreased expression of GSLs, galactosylceramide, sulfatides, and GM1 in particular.[120] The underlying mechanisms are not clear. The question remains whether at least some of these abnormalities are caused by the presence of antibodies against GM1 and other GSLs in the serum of patients with MS, which increase before the onset of disease, or by increased GSL-specific T-cell and B-cell reactivity.[121,122] This theory also may explain the presence of anti-GSL antibodies in the sera of AG/PDD-affected parrots.

Myelin stability and proper axonal function also depend on the interaction of GD1a and GT1b, the 2 most abundant GSLs in axonal membranes, with the myelin-associated glycoprotein (MAG), a sialic acid–binding protein. GD1a and GT1b are specific MAG ligands and their absence in the myelinated fibers results in aberrant neurofilament spacing and decreased axon caliber,[123] leading to axonal degeneration and demyelination of nerves in the nervous system.[124] Levels of GM1 at the plasma membrane of huntington disease (HD) cells correlate with cell susceptibility to apoptosis. Restoring normal GSL content in HD striatal cells by GM1 administration results in protection from cell death. Alternatively, decreasing the GM1 content of normal cells reproduces the susceptibility to apoptosis that is typical of HD. Therefore, GM1 at the plasma membrane of HD cells may play a role in the cell response to stress, perhaps by modulating the activation of pro-survival and/or pro-apoptotic pathways.[110] We have documented similar results in ganglia and peripheral nerves of AG/PDD-affected parrots, in which high serologic levels of anti-GM1 antibodies, which decrease the GM1 content in neuron plasma membranes, are related to major clinical signs of disease.[49] The disease process of AG/PDD involves inflammation of the nerve ganglia that exposes normally sequestered GSL proteins to the host immune system. Studies by Rossi and colleagues[45,46,94,95,97,125] have shown that the release of G 50 proteins from nerve ganglia produce pathologic lesions similar to that noted in the autoimmune neuropathy of GBS. Disease occurs when the host immune response is directed to these exposed proteins causing corresponding neurologic dysfunction. We suggest that AG/PDD is induced by an autoimmune mechanism similar to the pathogenesis of GBS, where GSLs act as major antigens. To confirm this theory, we challenged 6 young cockatiels intraperitoneally (IP) or orally with purified avian GSLs. One month after infection, 100% of IP-inoculated and 33% of orally challenged parrots developed neurologic and GI tract signs compatible with AG/PDD. Four of the birds demonstrated the classic lymphoplasmacytic ganglioneuritis in crop biopsies and all showed histopathological changes compatible with AG/PDD.[45]

We detected antibodies to nerve GSLs in the sera of AG/PDD-affected parrots, similar to those found in GBS. Quantification of such antibodies could be diagnostic for AG/PDD. Autoantibodies in the crop or gastrointestinal ganglia of parrots were observed by immunohistochemistry and immunoelectron microscopy. A robust antibody response to anti-GM1 GSL, strongly expressed in 15% of motor fibers, and 5% of sensory fibers of the GI tract, elicited an antibody-mediated phagocytosis and complement-induced damage of axons, with clinical signs of GI involvement, typical of AG/PDD.

This immune-mediated hypothesis is consistent with the autoimmune basis mentioned for various acute, postinfectious polyneuropathies associated with a wide range of viral and bacterial infections in animals and humans. In a recent epidemiologic survey, ABV was present in many but not all parrots with clinical AG/PDD.[126] This discrepancy may result from the fact that AG/PDD may be caused by ABV as well as by other, unrelated viruses or bacteria that induce an autoimmune ganglioneuritis. Undiscovered ABV strains with divergent genomes may exist that are not detected by current testing methods. Recently we tested parrot sera for Campylobacter jejuni lipo-oligosaccharide (LOS) and found a 93% cross-reactivity with sera from AG/PDD-affected parrots that had detectable anti-GSL antibodies. This "mistaken immune attack" may arise because the surface of C jejuni and other antigens contain lipopolysaccharides and LOS that resemble glycoconjugates of parrot nerve tissues.[127] Additionally, a recent report describes a peripheral ganglioneuritis, with incoordination, continuous tremors, regurgitation, dysarthria, diarrhea, lethargy, and weight loss in an African grey parrot (*P erithacus*) associated with an extended-spectrum beta-lactamase *Escherichia coli* infection.[128] Like GBS in humans, more agents may be discovered that induce an aberrant immune response that results in AG, This evidence of molecular mimicry reinforces the hypothesis that the antigen of the host (GSLs, cerebrosides, and myelin protein), delivered from infected tissues, triggers cross-reactive antibodies or T-cell activity that can lead to autoimmune ganglio-neuropathy.

Diagnosis

AG/PDD should be considered in the differential diagnosis of any bird exhibiting neurologic and/or gastrointestinal signs. Additionally, heart disease may be associated with AG/PDD. A presumptive diagnosis can be made based on the history, clinical signs, and radiographic evaluation of the digestive tract. Definitive diagnosis can be confirmed by demonstrating the characteristic histopathologic lesions in tissues from affected birds.

Plain and contrast radiography, and fluoroscopic evaluation of gastrointestinal motility, have been used for tentative antemortem diagnosis. Radiology and ultrasonography often reveal various degrees of enlargement, thinning, and/or impaction of the ingluvies, proventriculus, ventriculus, and proximal duodenum. The proventriculus is often severely dilated, filling the left side of the coelomic cavity. It often appears as a "J" shape causing the ventriculus to be displaced to the right and ventrally (see **Fig. 4**).[77] Dilatation and thinning of the wall of these organs may lead to impaction and rupture. Contrast studies often demonstrate prolonged transit times throughout the gastrointestinal tract.[40]

Clinical pathologic findings in AG/PDD are inconsistent and generally reflect the state of malnourishment, dehydration, and secondary infections that may occur with this disease. Serum chemistry profiles and complete blood counts are often normal, although a relative and absolute heterophilia, hypoproteinemia, anemia, gram-negative, and clostridial bacterial enteritis have been reported.[75] Gastrointestinal stasis predisposes to overgrowth of the digestive tract with yeast and gram-negative bacteria. Avian gastric yeast infections have also been associated with parrots that are at least suspect of AG/PDD (personal observation, SEO, 2017).

Antemortem diagnosis of AG/PDD can be confirmed by identification of the characteristic myenteric ganglioneuritis in biopsy samples of the crop, ventriculus, and adrenal gland.[52] Crop biopsy specimens should include a visible blood vessel/nerve complex. Unfortunately, not all birds with AG/PDD have crop lesions. The percentage of infiltration in the nerves of the crop is 40% to 76%.[32,39,52] Although reported to be an effective method of antemortem diagnosis, only approximately 76% of AG/PDD-affected birds have crop lesions and clinical biopsies are generally much smaller compared with those used in this study.[30,52] In practicality, crop biopsies are reported to be indicative of AG/PDD in only approximately 30% to 35% of cases.[30,32,52] Failure to observe lesions in a crop biopsy does not rule out the disease. It is suggested that biopsying the right cranial ventral aspect of the crop, making sure to include a blood vessel, may increase the probability of lesions being identified.[30]

Postmortem examination often reveals emaciation and the presence of a distended, impacted proventriculus and ventriculus. Thinning of the wall of these organs occurs and rupture of these organs may be present. Histologic examination of a wide range of tissues should be conducted on birds suspected of succumbing to AG/PDD. Tissues submitted should include the ingluvies, proventriculus, ventriculus, duodenum, adrenal gland, heart, spleen, and brain.

Differential Diagnoses

Tumors or papillomas of the crop, proventriculus, ventriculus, and intestines; ingestion of foreign bodies; macrorhabdosis; and parasitism can cause GI signs identical to those seen in AG/PDD.[10] Emptying of the proventriculus and ventriculus appears to be inhibited as long as the intestinal tract is distended. Inflammatory disease and neoplastic diseases of the ventriculus and proventriculus also can cause gastrointestinal stasis. Heavy metal poisoning is commonly associated with central nervous system signs but can cause GI stasis as well. Internal papillomatosis may result in a chronic wasting disease that resembles AG/PDD. AG/PDD should be considered as a differential in any bird with CNS disease. However, radiographically parrots with AG/PDD have a thinned mucosal wall compared with the other differential diagnoses and on fluoroscopy there is an abnormal mixing of the stomach contents with AG/PDD. Traumatic injuries; heavy metal poisoning; neoplasia; viral, bacterial, and fungal infections of the CNS; nutritional deficiencies; and hydrocephalus are additional diseases that can appear similar clinically.[10]

Avian Bornavirus Diagnostics

Polymerase chain reaction

The diagnosis of AG/PDD has traditionally been based on the identification of histologic lesions in biopsy or necropsy tissues. With the discovery of the association of ABV with AG/PDD, diagnostic testing has focused on RT-PCR for the detection of ABV RNA in affected birds. Antemortem detection of viral infection in the naturally or experimentally infected bird is, however, challenging. Urine, feces, and cloacal swabs are samples reportedly most likely to contain virus. However, a whole blood sample in combination with choanal/cloacal swabs may provide the greater sensitivity. Fecal swabs are less desirable, as RNAases and other degrading or inhibiting agents may rapidly degrade the viral RNA in these samples. Cloacal sampling, however, likely underestimates the prevalence of ABV infection. Intermittent urofecal shedding of ABV is described in both experimentally and naturally infected parrots, which can lead to a false-negative test result.[129,130] One research study recommended the use of feather calami for ABV RNA testing.[131] The consensus of opinion among most other researchers at the 2014 ABV Research Forum was that this was not an appropriate sample for accurate ABV testing.[9] It should be noted that there is no consistent or standardized method of testing among laboratories offering this service. Reported rates of ABV-positive tests among several university and commercial laboratories range from 3% to 33%. With only approximately 68% to 85% sequence identity among the known ABV genotypes, some assays may not be able to detect all ABV genotypes. Primers have been designed to target the nucleocapsid (N) gene, matrix (M) gene, phosphoprotein (P) gene, and polymerase (L) gene. Assays designed for detection of the M and immunodominant N gene sequences appear to have a similar high sensitivity.[54] Those for the L and P genes are generally less accurate. Both gel-based RT-PCR and real-time RT-PCR have been successfully used to detect ABV RNA. Real-time PCR assays appear to be the more sensitive of the 2 techniques.

Serology

Serologic assays have been used to detect ABV-exposed or infected birds. The indirect fluorescent antibody (IFA) assay is preferred by many investigators, particularly in Europe. Researchers in the United States tend to use the Western blot assay.[79,132]

Both appear to be sensitive and specific assays. They cannot, however, differentiate between diseased birds and healthy carriers. Not all birds shedding viral RNA are antibody positive.[46] The discrepancy among viral shedding, presence of antibodies, and clinical disease is now well recognized in parrots infected with ABV.[56,61,79] Viral shedding and presence of antibodies coincided in only one-fifth of the samples in a large study of captive psittacines.[56] In another study of free-ranging psittacines, 50% of ABV RNA-positive birds did not show antibodies against ABV by IFA.[11] Many apparently healthy birds may, however, be seronegative while, at the same time, shedding ABV in their feces.

In a large-scale study conducted in captive psittacine birds in Europe, 17% of the birds had detectable antibodies.[56] Widespread persistent asymptomatic infection with less common clinical disease is a consistent feature of bornavirus infections, and may be attributed to the lack of cytopathic effect of bornaviruses and their ability to escape recognition by the innate immune system.

Serologic testing for anti-GSL antibodies appears to more accurately detect clinically affected birds. Anti-GSL autoantibodies are used as markers of immune-mediated disease and are triggered by a variety of pathogens. High anti-GSL antibody levels were detected in 15.5% of 650 avian serum samples. Ninety-eight percent of birds that were symptomatic and histologically positive for AG/PDD had elevated serum anti-GSL antibody levels.[46,47] Anti-GSL antibody testing may be the preferred method to screen suspected birds for AG/PDD regardless of the etiologic cause.

Treatment

Medications

AG/PDD has historically been a fatal disease of psittacine birds with mortality approaching 100%. Even with appropriate supportive care, most birds succumb to progressive debilitation, starvation, secondary infections, or CNS disturbances. The ganglioneuritis and encephalomyelitis associated with AG/PDD is inflammatory in nature, the chronicity of which contributes to the progressive, debilitating nature of the disease. The rationale for a therapeutic approach was that diminishing this reaction was expected to lead to clinical improvement and possible resolution of clinical signs in affected birds. In 2002, it was demonstrated the resolution of clinical signs of AG/PDD by cyclooxygenase 2 (COX-2) inhibition.[63] Since this time, clinicians have recognized the early signs of avian ganglioneuritis and the variable ways it can present in a clinical setting. The use of preferential and selective COX-2 inhibitors has improved and extended the quality of life of affected birds. Celebrex has been used successfully in a number of avian patients as well as the use of robenacoxib by injection. The latter is important particularly in patients with delayed transit time of the GI tract. One study suggests that the use of meloxicam is contraindicated in avian patients with AG/PDD.[133] This study, however, infected a species with a large viral load, inducing severe disease, which is not normally encountered in nature. Clinical practitioners have anecdotally reported beneficial effects of meloxicam therapy.

Gastrointestinal prokinetic agents, such as cisapride (Propulsid; Janssen Pharmaceutica Inc., Titusville, NJ) and metoclopramide (Reglan; Schwarz Pharma, Seymour, IN) are helpful in improving transit in birds with GI tract involvement, especially early in the course of therapy. For those avian patients with alteration of normal proximal GI tract function, injectable metoclopramide is preferred, as normal uptake of drugs by oral administration is impaired.

Appropriate antibacterial and antifungal therapy should be instituted to control overgrowth of intestinal anaerobes, yeasts, and *Macrorhabdus ornithogaster* in these individuals. Gram stains/cultures of fresh feces may provide information regarding the gastrointestinal flora. This alteration of normal GI motility results in an altered intestinal microbiome. Probiotics and prebiotics (Sivoy, Rome, Italy) may prove helpful in restoring a normal intestinal environment. Omega fatty acids are also helpful in reducing inflammation both in the mucosal lining of the GI tract and nervous system tissues and clinically beneficial in affected birds.[134] Semi-elemental diets, such as Emeraid Omnivore and Carnivore (Lafeber Emeraid LLC, Cornell, IL) require minimal digestion and provide a readily absorbable source of essential nutrients and omega fatty acids. The liver is often exposed to bacterial showers from the abnormal intestinal environment in affected birds. Herbal supplements like milk thistle (Milk Thistle, Low Alcohol; Gaia Herbs, Brevard, NC) and ginger (Ginger Root, Certified Organic; Gaia Herbs, Brevard, NC) are helpful in reducing inflammation, preserving hepatic function, and improving GI tract transit.

Gabapentin (Neurontin; Pfizer, New York, NY) is increasingly being used in birds to help treat self-mutilation and to control the suspected neurogenic pain in some patients. It can be a useful adjunct in managing birds with AG.

Clinical signs in affected birds tend to increase with the onset of breeding activity. Reduction of the stress of elevated hormonal activity through the use of leuprolide acetate (Lupron Depot; AbbVie, Chicago, IL) or deslorelin implants (Suprelorin; Virbac Animal Health, Fort Worth, TX) can benefit patients as well. Off-label use of Suprelorin-F deslorelin acetate implants is prohibited by federal law in the United States because the product is not approved by the Food and Drug Administration, but legally marketed as an index drug.

Mammalian borna disease virus shows a high degree of sensitivity to ribavirin (Virazole; Valeant Pharmaceuticals International, Bridgewater, NJ), a ribonucleic analog that stops viral RNA synthesis. To date, the use of this and other antiviral agents in the treatment of ABV disease has not been rewarding or adequately researched.

Immunomodulation therapy through the use of *Mycobacterium bovis* extracts to redirected trafficking of activated antigen-specific CD4+ T cells to local inflammatory sites has been shown to modulate the initiation and progression of a Th1-mediated peripheral and CNS autoimmune disease. This researched group found significant improvement in clinically diseased birds when this approach was combined with selective anti–COX-2 therapy.[125]

Avian bornaviral vaccination

Research into the potential use of vaccination strategies to prevent ABV infection and disease is in its infancy. Using recombinant Newcastle disease virus (NDV) and modified vaccinia virus Ankara (MVA) vectors, engineered to express ABV phosphoprotein and nucleoprotein genes, Olbert and colleagues[135] were able to induce a bornavirus-specific humoral response in cockatiels (*N hollandicus*) and common canaries (*Serinus canaria forma domestica*). Shedding of bornavirus RNA and viral loads in tissue samples were significantly reduced in immunized birds after homologous bornavirus challenge infection. However, cockatiels still developed signs of AG/PDD and the vaccine failed to prevent viral persistence. Subsequent vaccination studies demonstrated that bornavirus replication was substantially blocked following homologous challenge infections.[136] Only 2 of 6 vaccinated birds had very low viral levels detectable in a few organs. Only one vaccinated bird developed mild AG/PDD-associated microscopic lesions. NDV and MVA vector vaccines can protect against invasive heterologous bornavirus challenge infections and subsequent AG/PDD. Implementation of these studies into a practical method of ABV/AG/PDD control may prove challenging. ABV has many strategies to evade the host immune system, leading to chronicity of infection. Additionally, research has shown that viral transmission via a nonparenteral route is difficult to nonexistent. Evidence does exist, however, that ABV is vertically transmitted through the egg. The effectiveness of vaccination on ABV-infected individuals has not been demonstrated. Practical application of vaccination strategies to control ABV infection and AG/PDD disease would be most useful if proven of benefit in these individuals.

With patience, perseverance, prolonged therapy, reduced stress, and attention to correction of secondary problems, quality and longevity of life in many ABV clinically affected birds can be significantly improved. Implementation of appropriate therapeutic plans, early in the course of clinical disease, are most productive. Therapies may be minimally effective in severely affected individuals.

FORMULARY

Celecoxib (Celebrex; Pfizer Inc., Mission, KS), initially 30 to 40 mg/kg divided twice a day by mouth, long term 15 to 20 mg/kg twice a day by mouth; 60 to 80 mg/kg divided twice a day by mouth for CNS involvement.

Robenacoxib (Onsior; Novartis Animal Health, North Ryde, NSW, Australia), 2 to 10 mg/kg intramuscularly weekly, and subsequently monthly.[97]

Meloxicam (Metacam; Boehringer Ingelheim Vetmedica Inc., St Joseph, MO), a preferential COX-2 inhibitor, not selective, 0.5 mg/kg IM, PO once daily. Oral form is formulated for canine species and may have reduced bioavailability in avian species; one clinical trial has shown its use exacerbates signs of clinical disease in ABV-infected cockatiels.[133]

Gabapentin (Neurontin; Pfizer, New York, NY) 10 to 25 mg/kg twice a day by mouth up to 50 mg/kg twice a day by mouth in self-mutilating birds (Cathy Johnson-Delaney, written communication, 2015).

REFERENCES

1. Clark FD. Proventricular dilatation syndrome in large psittacine birds. Avian Dis 1984;28(3):813–5.
2. Gerlach H. Uber das Sog. "Macaw wasting syndrome." Vortrag, 4. Arbeitstagung der Zootierarzte im deutschsprachigen Raum. Munster, Germany. November 24–25, 1984.
3. Graham DL. Infiltrative splanchnic neuropathy, a component of the "wasting macaw" complex. Proc. Int. Conf. on Avian Med. Toronto (Canada), June 20–23, 1984. p. 275.
4. Hughes PE. The pathology of myenteric ganglioneuritis, psittacine encephalomyelitis, proventricular dilatation of psittacines, and macaw wasting syndrome. Proc 33rd West Poult Dis Conf. Davis (CA), March 4–6, 1984. p. 85–87.
5. Phalen DN. An outbreak of psittacine proventricular dilatation syndrome (PPDS) in a private collection of birds and an atypical form of PPDS in a nanday conure. Proc Annu Conf Assoc Avian Vet. Miami (FL), June 16–22, 1986. p. 27–34.
6. Ridgway RA, Gallerstein GA. Proventricular dilatation in psittacines. Proc 4th Annu Meet Assoc Avian Vet. San Diego (CA), June 1–5, 1983. p. 228–230.
7. Woerpel, RW, Rosskopf WJ. Clinical and pathological features of macaw wasting disease (proventricular dilatation syndrome). Proc 33rd Western Poultry Dis Conf. Davis (CA), February 27–29, 1984. p. 89–90.
8. Woerpel, RW, Rosskopf WJ. Proventricular dilatation and wasting syndrome: myenteric ganglioneurtitis and encephalomyelitis of psittacines; an update. Proc Int Conf on Avian Med. Toronto (Canada), June 20–23, 1984. p. 25–28.
9. Avian Bornavirus Research Forum. Association of Avian Vet Conference. New Orleans (LA), August 2–6, 2014.

10. Schmidt RE, Reavill DR, Phalen DN. Pathology of pet and aviary birds. Ames (IA): Iowa State Press; 2003. p. 47–55.
11. Encinas-Nagel N, Enderlein D, Piepenbring A, et al. Avian bornavirus in free-ranging psittacine birds, Brazil. Emerg Infect Dis 2014;20(12):2103–6.
12. Daoust PY, Julian RJ, Yason CV, et al. Proventricular impaction associated with nonsuppurative encephalomyelitis and ganglioneuritis in two Canada geese. J Wildl Dis 1991;27(3):513–7.
13. Gregory CR, Ritchie BW, Latimer KS, et al. Progress in understanding proventricular dilatation disease. Proc Annu Conf Assoc Avian Vet. Portland (OR), August 30-September 1, 2000. p. 269–275.
14. Perpiñán D, Fernández-Bellon H, López C, et al. Lymphoplasmacytic myenteric, subepicardial, and pulmonary ganglioneuritis in four nonpsittacine birds. J Avian Med Surg 2007;21(3):210–4.
15. Shivaprasad HL. Proventricular dilatation disease in a peregrine falcon (*Falco peregrinus*). Proc Annu Conf Assoc Avian Vet. Monterey (CA), August 8–12, 2005. p. 107–108.
16. Weissebock H, Bakonyi T, Sekulin K, et al. Avian bornaviruses in psittacine birds from Europe and Australia with proventricular dilatation disease. Emerg Infect Dis 2009;15:1453–9.
17. Cazayoux Vice CA. Myocarditis as a component of psittacine proventricular dilatation syndrome in a Patagonian conure. Avian Dis 1992;36(4):1117–9.
18. Breazile JE, Kuenzel WJ. Systema nervosus centrale. In: Baumel JJ, editor. Handbook of avian anatomy: nomina anatomica avium. Cambridge: Nuttall Ornithological Club, No. 23; 1993. p. 493–554.
19. Carpenter MB. The medulla. In: Human neuroanatomy. 7th edition. Baltimore (MD): Williams & Wilkins; 1976. p. 309–11.
20. De LaHunta A. Lower motor neuron–general visceral efferent system. In: Veterinary neuroanatomy and clinical neurology. Philadelphia: WB Saunders; 1977. p. 122–4.
21. Tizard I, Shivaprasad HL, Guo J, et al. The pathogenesis of proventricular dilatation disease. Anim Health Res Rev 2016;17(2):110–26.
22. Sanders KM, Koh SD, Ward SM. Interstitial cells of Cajal as pacemakers in the gastrointestinal tract. Annu Rev Physiol 2006;68:307–43.
23. Dziuk HE, Duke GE. Cineradiographic studies of the gastric motility in turkeys. Am J Physiol 1972;222:159–66.
24. McLelland J. Digestive system. In: King AS, McLelland J, editors. Form and function in birds. London: Academic Press; 1989. p. 69–181.
25. Chaplin SB, Duke GE. Effect of denervation of the myenteric plexus on gastroduodenal motility in turkeys. Am J Physiol 1990;259:G481–9.
26. Torihashi S, Horisawa M, Watanabe Y. c-Kit immunoreactive interstitial cells in the human gastrointestinal tract. J Auton Nerv Syst 1999;75:38–50.
27. Hirst GD, Beckett EA, Sanders KM, et al. Regional variation in contribution of myenteric and intramuscular interstitial cells of Cajal to generation of slow waves in mouse gastric antrum. J Physiol 2002;540:1003–12.
28. Mazet B, Raynier C. Interstitial cells of Cajal in the guinea pig gastric antrum: distribution and regional density. Cell Tissue Res 2004;316:23–34.
29. Pavlov VA, Tracey KJ. The vagus nerve and the inflammatory reflex linking immunity and metabolism. Nat Rev Endocrinol 2012;8:743–54.
30. Andersson U, Tracey KJ. Reflex principles of immunological homeostasis. Annu Rev Immunol 2011;30:313–35.
31. Tracey KJ. The inflammatory reflex. Nature 2002;420:853–9.

32. Berhane Y, Smith D, Newman S, et al. Peripheral neuritis in psittacine birds with proventricular dilatation disease. Avian Pathol 2001;30:563–70.

33. Korbel R, Rinder M. Ophthalmological findings in birds affected with PDD. Proc 11th Eur Assoc Avian Vet Conf. Seattle (WA), August 6–12, 2011. p. 193.

34. Philadelpho NA, Rubbenstroth D, Guimara MB, et al. Survey of bornaviruses in pet psittacines in Brazil reveals a novel parrot bornavirus. Vet Microbiol 2014; 174:584–90.

35. Graham DL. Wasting/proventricular dilatation disease. A pathologist's view. Proc Annu Conf Assoc Avian Vet. Chicago (IL), September 23–28, 1991. p. 43–44.

36. Reavill D and Schmidt R. Lesions of the proventriculus/ventriculus of pet birds: 1640 cases. Proc Annu Conf Assoc Avian Vet. Providence (RI), August 6–9, 2007. p. 89–93.

37. Gancz AY, Kistler AL, Greninger AL, et al. Experimental induction of proventricular dilatation disease in cockatiels (*Nymphicus hollandicus*) inoculated with brain homogenates containing avian bornavirus 4. Virol J 2009;6:11.

38. Rossi G, Galosi L, Dahlhausen B, et al. Unusual and severe lesions of proventricular dilatation disease in lories. In: Proceedings of the 3rd ICARE, International Conference on Avian Herpetological and Exotic Mammal Medicine. Venice (Italy), March 25–29, 2017. p. 663.

39. Shivaprasad HL. Spectrum of lesions (pathology) of proventricular dilation syndrome. Proc Annu Conf Assoc Avian Vet. Nashville (TN), August 31–September 4, 1995. p. 505–506.

40. Gerlach H. Macaw wasting disease–a four-year study on clinical case history, epizootiology, analysis of species, diagnosis, and differential diagnosis, microbiological and virological results. Proc Annu Conf Assoc Avian Vet. Chicago (IL), September 23–28, 1991. p. 377–400.

41. Doneley RJT, Miller RI, Fanning TE. Proventricular dilatation disease: an emerging exotic disease of parrots in Australia. Aust Vet J 2007;85:119–23.

42. Mannl A, Gerlach H, Leipold R. Neuropathic gastric dilatation in Psittaciformes. Avian Dis 1987;31:214–21.

43. Steinmetz A, Pees M, Schmidt V, et al. Blindness as a sign of proventricular dilatation disease in a grey parrot (*Psittacus erithacus erithacus*). J Small Anim Pract 2008;49(12):660–2.

44. de Araujo JL, Tizard I, Guo J, et al. Are anti-ganglioside antibodies associated with proventricular dilatation disease in birds? PeerJ 2017;5:e3144.

45. Rossi G, Crosta L, Ceccherelli R, et al. New evidence in AG/PDD pathogenesis: can ganglioside sensitization satisfy Koch's postulates? Proc Eur Assoc Avian Vet. Antwerp (Belgium), March 17–21, 2009. p. 155.

46. Rossi G, Ceccherelli R, Crosta L, et al. Anti-ganglioside specific auto-antibodies in ganglia of PDD-affected parrots. Proc 11th Eur AAV Conf, 1st Sci ECZM Meeting. Madrid (Spain), April 26–30, 2011. p. 177–178.

47. Pesaro S, Crosta L, Bertoni P, et al. Anti-ganglioside antibodies production as a theory of PDD pathogenesis. Proc Eur Assoc Avian Vet. Antwerp (Belgium), March 17–21, 2009. p. 89.

48. Leonardi E, Girlando S, Serio G, et al. PCNA and Ki67 expression in breast carcinoma: correlations with clinical and biological variables. J Clin Pathol 1992;45:416–9.

49. Moldovan GL, Pfander B, Jentsch S. PCNA, the maestro of the replication fork. Cell 2007;129(4):665–79.

50. Chao CY, Zheng YP, Cheing GL. The association between skin blood flow and edema on epidermal thickness in the diabetic foot. Diabetes Technol Ther 2012;14(7):602–9.

51. Tavee J, Zhou L. Small fiber neuropathy: a burning problem. Cleve Clin J Med 2009;76(5):297–305.
52. Kistler AL, Gancz A, Clubb S, et al. Recovery of divergent avian bornaviruses from cases of proventricular dilatation disease: identification of a candidate etiologic agent. Virol J 2008;5:88.
53. Honkavuori KS, Shivaprasad HL, Williams BL, et al. Novel borna virus in psittacine birds with proventricular dilatation disease. Emerg Infect Dis 2008;14:1883–6.
54. Lierz M, Hafez HM, Honkavuori KS, et al. Anatomical distribution of avian bornavirus in parrots, its occurrence in clinically healthy birds and ABV antibody detection. Avian Pathol 2009;38:491–6.
55. Gough RE, Drury SE, Harcourt-Brown NH, et al. Virus-like particles associated with macaw wasting disease. Vet Rec 1996;139:24.
56. Heffels-Redmann U, Enderlein D, Herzog S, et al. Occurrence of avian bornavirus infection in captive psittacines in various European countries and its association with proventricular dilatation disease. Avian Pathol 2011;40:419–26.
57. Piepenbring AK, Enderlein D, Herzog S, et al. Pathogenesis of avian bornavirus in experimentally infected cockatiels. Emerg Infect Dis 2012;18:234–41.
58. Gray P, Hoppes S, Suchodolski P, et al. Use of avian bornavirus isolates to induce proventricular dilatation disease in conures. Emerg Infect Dis 2010; 16(3):473–9.
59. Kuhn JH, Dürrwald R, Bào Y, et al. Taxonomic reorganization of the family Bornaviridae. Arch Virol 2015;160:621–32.
60. Rubbenstroth D, Rinder M, Kaspers B, et al. Efficient isolation of avian bornaviruses (ABV) from naturally infected psittacine birds and identification of a new ABV genotype from a salmon-crested cockatoo (Cacatua moluccensis). Vet Microbiol 2012;161(1–2):36–42.
61. Piepenbring AK, Enderlein D, Herzog S, et al. Parrot bornavirus (PaBV)-2 isolate causes different disease patterns in cockatiels than PaBV-4. Avian Pathol 2016; 45(2):156–68.
62. Rinder M, Ackermann A, Kempf H, et al. Broad tissue and cell tropism of avian bornavirus in parrots with proventricular dilatation disease. J Virol 2009;83: 5401–7.
63. Reuter A, Ackermann A, Kothlow S, et al. Avian bornaviruses escape recognition by the innate immune system. Viruses 2010;2:927–38.
64. Lierz M. Avian Borna virus research at the free University of Berlin. Presented at the research Forum of the 10th European AAV Conf. Antwerp (Belgium), March 17–21, 2009.
65. Herzog S, Enderlein D, Heffels-Redmann U, et al. Indirect immunofluorescence assay for intra vitam diagnostic of avian Borna virus infection in psittacine birds. J Clin Microbiol 2010;48(6):2282–4.
66. Dahlhausen RD, Orosz SE. Avian borna virus infection rates in domestic psittacine birds. Proc Annu Conf Assoc Avian Vet. San Diego (CA), August 1–5, 2010. p. 49.
67. Rubbenstroth D, Rinder M, Stein M, et al. Avian bornaviruses are widely distributed in canary birds (Serinus canaria f. domestica). Vet Microbiol 2013;165:287–95.
68. Payne S, Covaleda L, Jianhua G, et al. Detection and characterization of a distinct bornavirus lineage from healthy Canada geese (Branta canadensis). J Virol 2011;85(22):12053–6.
69. Rubbenstroth D, Brosinski K, Rinder M, et al. No contact transmission of avian bornavirus in experimentally infected cockatiels (Nymphicus hollandicus) and domestic canaries (Serinus canaria forma domestica). Vet Microbiol 2014; 172(1–2):146–56.

70. Kistler AL, Smith JM, Greninger AL, et al. Analysis of naturally occurring avian bornavirus infection and transmission during an outbreak of proventricular dilatation disease among captive psittacine birds. J Virol 2010;84:2176–9.

71. Heckmann J, Enderlein D, Piepenbring A, et al. Investigation of different infection routes of parrot bornavirus in cockatiels. Avian Dis 2017;61(1):90–5.

72. Heffels-Redmann U, Enderlein D, Herzog S, et al. Follow-up investigations on different courses of natural avian bornavirus infections in Psittacines. Avian Dis 2012;56:153–9.

73. Rubbenstroth D, Schmidt V, Rinder M, et al. Phylogenetic analysis supports horizontal transmission as a driving force of the spread of avian bornaviruses. PLoS One 2016;11(8):e0160936.

74. Kerski A, de Kloet AH, de Kloet SR. Vertical transmission of avian bornavirus in Psittaciformes: avian bornavirus RNA and anti-avian bornavirus antibodies in eggs, embryos, and hatchlings obtained from infected sun conures (Aratinga solstitialis). Avian Dis 2012;56:471–8.

75. Lierz M, Piepenbring A, Herden C, et al. Vertical transmission of avian bornavirus in psittacines. Emerg Infect Dis 2011;17(12):2390–1.

76. Monaco E, Hoppes S, Guo J, et al. The detection of avian bornavirus within psittacine eggs. J Avian Med Surg 2012;26:144–8.

77. Phalen DN. Implications of viruses in clinical disorders. In: Harrison GJ, Lightfoot TL, editors. Clinical avian medicine. Palm Beach (FL): Spix Publishing; 2006. p. 721–46.

78. Kranz JB, Escandon P, Musser JMB. Environmental stability of avian Bornavirus: pH and drying. Proc ExoticsCon. San Antonio (TX), August 29–September 2, 2015. p. 89.

79. Lierz M, Piepenbring A, Heffels-Redmann U, et al. Experimental infection of cockatiels with different avian bornavirus genotype. Proc Annu Conf Assoc Avian Vet. Louisville (KY), August 12–15, 2012. p. 9–10.

80. Payne S, Shivaprasad HL, Mirhosseinia N, et al. Unusual and severe lesions of proventricular dilatation disease in cockatiels (Nymphicus hollandicus) acting as healthy carriers of avian bornavirus (ABV) and subsequently infected with a virulent strain of ABV. Avian Pathol 2011;40(1):15–22.

81. Mirhosseini N, Gray PL, Hoppes S, et al. Proventricular dilatation disease in cockatiels (Nymphicus hollandicus) after infection with a genotype 2 avian bornavirus. J Avian Med Surg 2011;25(3):199–204.

82. Payne SL, Delnatte P, Guo J, et al. Birds and bornaviruses. Anim Health Res Rev 2012;13(2):145–56.

83. Gray P, Villanueva I, Mirhosseini et al. Experimental infection of birds with avian bornavirus. Proc Annu Conf Assoc Avian Vet. Milwaukee (WI), August 10–13, 2009. p. 7–8.

84. Hoppes SM, Tizard I, Shivaprasad HL. Avian bornavirus and proventricular dilatation disease: diagnostics, pathology, prevalence, and control. Vet Clin North Am Exot Anim Pract 2013;16(2):339–55.

85. Okamoto M, Hagiwara K, Kamitani W, et al. Experimental vertical transmission of Borna disease virus in the mouse. Arch Virol 2003;148(8):1557–68.

86. Rott R, Herzog S, Richt J, et al. Immune-mediated pathogenesis of Borna disease. Zentralbl Bakteriol Mikrobiol Hyg A 1988;270(1–2):295–301.

87. Stitz L, Soeder D, Deschl U, et al. Inhibition of immune-mediated meningoencephalitis in persistently borna disease virus-infected rats by cyclosporine A. J Immunol 1989;143(12):4250–6.

88. Hallensleben W, Schwemmle M, Hausmann J, et al. Borna disease virus-induced neurological disorder in mice: infection of neonates results in immuno-pathology. J Virol 1998;72(5):4379–86.
89. Matsumoto Y, Hayashi Y, Omori H, et al. Bornavirus closely associates and seg-regates with host chromosomes to ensure persistent intranuclear infection. Cell Host Microbe 2012;11(5):492–503.
90. Stitz L, Dietzschold B, Carbone KM. Immunopathogenesis of Borna disease. Curr Top Microbiol Immunol 1995;190:75–92.
91. Stitz L, Bilzer T, Planz O. The immunopathogenesis of borna disease virus infec-tion. Front Biosci 2002;7:d541–55.
92. Schwemmle M, Billich C. The use of peptide arrays for the characterization of monospecific antibody repertoires from polyclonal sera of psychiatric patients suspected of infection by borna disease virus. Mol Divers 2004;8(3):247–50.
93. Baur K, Rauer M, Richter K, et al. Antiviral CD8 T cells recognize borna disease virus antigen transgenically expressed in either neurons or astrocytes. J Virol 2008;82(6):3099–108.
94. Rossi G, Crosta L, Pesaro S. Parrot proventricular dilation disease. Vet Rec 2008;163:310.
95. Rossi G, Enderlein D, Herzog S, et al. Comparison of anti-ganglioside anti-bodies and anti-ABV antibodies in psittacines. Proc 11th Eur AAV Conf, 1st Sci ECZM Meeting. Madrid (Spain), April 26–30, 2011. p. 187–189.
96. Pesaro S, Crosta L, Bertoni P, et al. Anti-ganglioside antibodies production like a theory for PDD's pathogenesis. Proc 11th Eur AAV Conf, 1st Sci ECZM Meeting. Madrid (Spain), April 26–30, 2011. p. 89.
97. Rossi G, Crosta L, Ceccherelli R, et al, PDD: our point of view after 7 years of research. Proc Annu Conf Assoc Avian Vet. Louisville (KY), August 12–15, 2012. p. 79–80.
98. Casteleyn C, Doom M, Lambrechts E, et al. Location of gut associated lymphoid tissue in the 3 month old chicken: a review. Avian Pathol 2010;39:143–50.
99. Hoppes S, Gray PL, Payne S, et al. The isolation, pathogenesis, diagnosis, transmission, and control of avian bornavirus and proventricular dilatation dis-ease. Vet Clin North Am Exot Anim Pract 2010;13(3):495–508.
100. Walport MJ. Complement. First of two parts. N Engl J Med 2001;344(14): 1058–66.
101. Walport MJ. Complement. Second of two parts. N Engl J Med 2001;344(15): 1140–4.
102. Pasinetti GM, Johnson SA, Rozovsky I, et al. Complement C1qB and C4 mRNAs responses to lesioning in rat brain. Exp Neurol 1992;118(2):117–25.
103. Frank MM, Fries LF. The role of complement in inflammation and phagocytosis. Immunol Today 1991;12(9):322–6.
104. Müller-Eberhard HJ. The membrane attack complex of complement. Annu Rev Immunol 1986;4:503–28.
105. Dietzschold B, Schwaeble W, Schäfer MK, et al. Expression of C1q, a subcom-ponent of the rat complement system, is dramatically enhanced in brains of rats with either borna disease or experimental allergic encephalomyelitis. J Neurol Sci 1995;130(1):11–6.
106. McGeer PL, Akiyama H, Itagaki S, et al. Immune system response in Alzheimer's disease. Can J Neurol Sci 1989;16(4 Suppl):516–27.
107. Yamada T, Akiyama H, McGeer PL. Complement-activated oligodendroglia: a new pathogenic entity identified by immunostaining with antibodies to human complement proteins C3d and C4d. Neurosci Lett 1990;112(2–3):161–6.

108. Bordin S, Ghebrehiwet B, Page RC. Participation of C1q and its receptor in adherence of human diploid fibroblast. J Immunol 1990;145(8):2520–6.

109. Guan EN, Burgess WH, Robinson SL. Phagocytic cell molecules that bind the collagen-like region of C1q. Involvement in the C1q-mediated enhancement of phagocytosis. J Biol Chem 1991;266(30):20345–55.

110. Koprowski H, Zheng YM, Heber-Katz E, et al. In vivo expression of inducible nitric oxide synthase in experimentally induced neurologic diseases. Proc Natl Acad Sci USA 1993;90(7):3024–7.

111. Rauer M, Götz J, Schuppli D, et al. Transgenic mice expressing the nucleoprotein of Borna disease virus in either neurons or astrocytes: decreased susceptibility to homotypic infection and disease. J Virol 2004;78(7):3621–32.

112. Asbury AK, Arnason BG, Adams RD. The inflammatory lesion in idiopathic polyneuritis. Its role in pathogenesis. Medicine (Baltimore) 1969;48(3):173–215.

113. Griffin JW, Li CY, Macko C, et al. Neurocytol. Early nodal changes in the acute motor axonal neuropathy pattern of the Guillain-Barré syndrome. J Neurocytol 1996;25(1):33–51.

114. Griffin JW, Li CY, Ho TW, et al. Pathology of the motor-sensory axonal Guillain-Barré syndrome. Ann Neurol 1996;39(1):17–28.

115. Prineas JW, Wright RG. The fine structure of peripheral nerve lesions in a virus-induced demyelinating disease in fowl (Marek's disease). Lab Invest 1972; 26(5):548–57.

116. Staeheli P, Rinder M, Kaspers B. Avian bornavirus associated with fatal disease in psittacine birds. J Virol 2010;84(13):6269–75.

117. Tettamanti G. Ganglioside/glycosphingolipid turnover: new concepts. Glycoconj J 2004;20(5):301–17.

118. Sonnino S, Chigorno V. Ganglioside molecular species containing C18- and C20-sphingosine in mammalian nervous tissues and neuronal cell cultures. Biochim Biophys Acta 2000;1469(2):63–77.

119. Labasque M, Faivre-Sarrailh C. GPI-anchored proteins at the node of Ranvier. FEBS Lett 2010;584(9):1787–92.

120. Howell OW, Palser A, Polito A, et al. Disruption of neurofascin localization reveals early changes preceding demyelination and remyelination in multiple sclerosis. Brain 2006;129:3173–85.

121. Pender MP, Csurhes PA, Wolfe NP, et al. Increased circulating T cell reactivity to GM3 and GQ1b gangliosides in primary progressive multiple sclerosis. J Clin Neurosci 2003;10:63–6.

122. Valentino P, Labate A, Nisticò R, et al. Anti-GM1 antibodies are not associated with cerebral atrophy in patients with multiple sclerosis. Mult Scler 2009;15: 114–5.

123. Pan B, Fromholt SE, Hess EJ, et al. Myelin-associated glycoprotein and complementary axonal ligands, gangliosides, mediate axon stability in the CNS and PNS: neuropathology and behavioral deficits in single-and double-null mice. Exp Neurol 2005;195(1):208–17.

124. Sheikh KA, Sun J, Liu Y, et al. Mice lacking complex gangliosides develop Wallerian degeneration and myelination defects. Proc Natl Acad Sci USA 1999; 96(13):7532–7.

125. Rossi G, Pesaro S, Ceccherelli R, et al. Update and perspectives on PDD treatment; results of three years of immunomodulating therapy. Proc 1st International Conference on Avian, Herpetological, and Exotic Mammal Medicine. Weisbaden (Germany), April 20–26, 2013. p. 351.

126. Shivaprasad HL. Proventricular dilatation disease but negative for avian bornavirus in raptors: a toucan and a mousebird. Proc Annu Conf Assoc Avian Vet. Portland (OR), August 27–September 1, Portland (OR), August 27–September 1, 2016. p. 97.
127. Rossi G, Piccinini A, Heikema AP, et al. Camplyobacter jejuni and proventricular dilatation disease in parrots: there may be a correlation? Proceedings of International Conference on Avian, Herpetological, and Exotic Mammal Medicine. Paris, France, 2015. p. 390.
128. Bert E. A case of PDD associated to ESBL *Escherichia coli* infection in an African grey parrot (*Psittacus E. erithacus*). Proc 3rd International Conference on Avian, Herpetological, and Exotic Mammal Medicine. Venice (Italy). March 25–29, 2017.
129. Raghav R, Taylor M, Delay J, et al. Avian bornavirus is present in many tissues of psittacine birds with histopathologic evidence of proventricular dilatation disease. J Vet Diagn Invest 2010;22:495–508.
130. Heatley JJ, Villalobos AR. Avian bornavirus in the urine of infected birds. Vet Med Res Rep 2012;3:19–23.
131. de Kloet AH, Kerski A, de Kloet SR. Diagnosis of avian bornavirus infection in psittaciformes by serum antibody detection and reverse transcription polymerase chain reaction assay using feather calami. J Vet Diagn Invest 2011;23(3): 421–9.
132. Villanueva I, Gray P, Mirhosseini N, et al. The diagnosis of proventricular dilatation disease: use of a Western blot assay to detect antibodies against avian borna virus. Vet Microbiol 2010;143:196–201.
133. Hoppes S, Heatley J, Guo J, et al. Meloxicam treatment in cockatiels (*Nymphicus hollandicus*) infected with avian bornavirus. J Exot Pet Med 2013;22:275–9.
134. Clubb SL. Clinical management of psittacine birds affected with proventricular dilatation disease. Proc Annu Conf Assoc Avian Vet. San Antonio (TX), August 29–September 2, 2015. p. 85–90.
135. Olbert M, Römer-Oberdörfer A, Herden C, et al. Viral vector vaccines expressing nucleoprotein and phosphoprotein genes of avian bornaviruses ameliorate homologous challenge infections in cockatiels and common canaries. Sci Rep 2016;6:36840.
136. Runge S, Olbert M, Herden C, et al. Viral vector vaccines protect cockatiels from inflammatory lesions after heterologous parrot bornavirus 2 challenge infection. Vaccine 2017;35(4):557–63.

Clinical Signs, Diagnosis, and Treatment of *Encephalitozoon cuniculi* Infection in Rabbits

Frank Künzel, DVM, Dr, Priv Doz, DECZM (Small Mammal)[a],[*],
Peter G. Fisher, DVM, DABVP (Exotic Companion Mammal Practice)[b]

KEYWORDS

- Encephalitozoonosis • *Encephalitozoon cuniculi* • Neurologic disorders
- Vestibular dysfunction • Clinical signs • Diagnosis • Rabbit • Microsporidia

KEY POINTS

- Central vestibular dysfunction caused by *Encephalitozoon cuniculi* frequently mimics the condition of a peripheral disorder.
- A negative antibody titer rules out *E cuniculi* as the cause of present clinical signs.
- Cerebrospinal fluid analysis including polymerase chain reaction is considered an inappropriate diagnostic method for in vivo diagnosis of encephalitozoonosis.
- The usefulness of glucocorticoid anti-inflammatories in the treatment of encephalitozoonosis is called into question.
- Encouraging activity early in the course of disease and adding in therapeutic exercise may represent the most important part of therapy in rabbits with vestibular dysfunction associated with encephalitozoonosis.

INTRODUCTION/BIOLOGY OF *ENCEPHALITOZOON CUNICULI*
Classification and Cell Structure

Encephalitozoon cuniculi is a mammalian microsporidian pathogen with worldwide distribution that may infect various species of mammals, including humans. The phylogenetic origin of microsporidia has been a consistent matter of debate because they possess many unique features that make them difficult to compare with other organisms. Microsporidia were originally thought to lack mitochondria and thus considered

Disclosure Statement: The authors have nothing to disclose.
[a] Clinical Department of Small Animals and Horses, University of Veterinary Medicine Vienna, Veterinaerplatz 1, 1210 Vienna, Austria; [b] Pet Care Veterinary Hospital, 5201 Virginia Beach Boulevard, Virginia Beach, VA 23462, USA
* Corresponding author.
E-mail address: frank.kuenzel@vetmeduni.ac.at

to be very basic eukaryotes. However, small and highly reduced mitochondria, known as mitosomes, have been identified at the cell organelle level and are now considered to be an important differentiating characteristic of the microsporidia. The discovery of a gene for this mitochondrial-type chaperone combined with phylogenetic analysis of multiple gene sequences supports a relationship between the microsporida and atypical fungi with extreme host cell dependency.[1–3] In addition, microsporidial spores retain fungal elements, including fungal proteins, such as tubulins, trehalose, and chitin.[3] The exact branching position within the fungal tree has not been completely clarified; however, gene sequencing supports a relationship with the ascomycete and basidiomycete clade.[1]

Microsporidia produce environmentally resistant spores and survive only by living in other cells. Microsporidia possess a unique method of infecting other cells that involves a specialized extrusion apparatus known as the polar tube or filament. This coiled tube is joined to an anchoring disc at the apical part of the spore and is a key diagnostic structure used for identification. The polar tube serves as a sporal invasive apparatus whereby a change in pH or osmotic pressure results in an explosive uncoiling of the polar tube with subsequent discharge of infectious sporoplasm either directly into the host cell or after spore phagocytosis by the host cell. In the first method of infection, polar tube uncoiling results in direct invagination of the host cell plasma membrane giving rise to transfer of sporoplasm via creation of a parsitophorous vacuole (PV) where E cuniculi spends its entire intracellular life cycle.[3] Alternatively, this transfer of nucleus-containing sporoplasm may occur after host cell phagocytosis and subsequent polar tube discharge and uptake of sporoplasm by host-cell phagosomes.[4] It has been suggested that germination out of phagosomes is limited and does not significantly contribute to E cuniculi infection.[3]

Life Cycle and Pathogenesis

E cuniculi has a direct life cycle with both horizontal and vertical (transplacental) transmission. In rabbits, postnatal transmission often occurs within 6 weeks from an infected dam or contact with other infected animals.[5] Spores, measuring 1.5 × 2.5 μm, are either ingested or inhaled as the infectious stage of E cuniculi, with oral ingestion of spores from infected rabbit urine being the most common source of infection. Spores can be found in the urine 1 month after infection and are excreted in large numbers up to 2 months after infection.[6] E cuniculi spores can survive outside the host for up to 6 weeks at 72°F (22°C). Shedding of spores is essentially terminated by 3 months after infection with very intermittent shedding of small amounts of spores by the infected rabbit thereafter. Following germination via the polar tube extrusion process described above, the microsporidia undergo a proliferative phase during merogony. Morphologically simple structured cells (meronts) replicate by binary or multiple division within host cell parasitophorous vacuoles, where they are found attached and closely aligned with the PV membrane. Initial target organs for infection include those with high blood flow such as the lungs, liver, and kidney, with infection of nervous tissue occurring later in the course of the disease.[7] Further differentiation of meronts into sporonts and later into mature spores (sporogony) results in the development of the distinctive polar filament and a rigid spore wall. With time, the PV or pseudocyst becomes overcrowded and ruptures, resulting in spore release. Cell rupture is associated with an inflammatory response, and most immunocompetent rabbits develop chronic, subclinical infections in a balanced host-parasite relationship associated with granulomatous lesions primarily affecting the brain, kidney, or eyes. A wide range of tissues may show morphologic lesions; however, in general, these histologic alterations are not associated with clinical disease.

As the host animal ages and becomes less immune competent, *E cuniculi* is occasionally associated with clinical disease in pet rabbits, most commonly neurologic disease. Encephalitozoonosis seems to be a widespread disease in rabbits with reports of infection found in 50% to 75% of conventional rabbit colonies (**Fig. 1**).[8]

Encephalitozoon cuniculi in Other Mammals and Humans

E cuniculi is the most commonly reported microsporidian of nonhuman mammals.[9] Other than rabbits, symptomatic infection appears to be rare. Three strains of *E cuniculi* have been characterized: strain I (karyotypes A,B,C) reported in rabbits, mice, and humans; strain II (karyotype F) in blue foxes, mice, and cats; and strain III (karyotypes D, E) isolated from domestic dogs and humans.[9] A former undescribed strain has recently been identified in a renal-transplant recipient with a disseminated *E cuniculi* infection and in cats with *E cuniculi*–associated ocular lesions.[10,11] Unclassified strains have been reported in a wide host range of mammals, including rats, guinea pigs, hamsters, horses, cows, mink, and nonhuman primates.[9] Several reports have identified *E cuniculi* in asymptomatic laboratory rats and guinea pigs based on histopathologic identification of the organism in the central nervous system (CNS) on necropsy and/or serology.[12–14] A new *E cuniculi* isolate, identified in free-ranging rats, was characterized as strain II based on the recombinant DNA internal spacer sequence.[15] Western blot analysis of this isolate revealed slight differences to other strain II isolates originating from laboratory mice and farmed blue foxes. This new isolate caused disseminated infection in liver and lungs upon oral inoculation of Brown Norway rats and was transmitted to sentinel rats.[15] In dogs, infection is most common in pups born to infected dams, with clinical signs being primarily neurologic: depression, ataxia, blindness, and seizures.[16,17] In one case series of 19 dogs (all puppies), histopathologic evaluation showed lesions typical of encephalitis and nephritis with molecular analysis confirming association with infectious organisms identified as *E cuniculi* strain III in 13 cases.[17] Worldwide serologic studies have been conducted on dogs with specific antibodies ranging from 8% to 38%.[16] *E cuniculi* may infect domestic cats with both meningoencephalitis and interstitial nephritis being reported, although these infections are rare and poorly studied. However, in the last few years, several cases of anterior uveitis and cataract have been documented in felids associated with *E cuniculi*.[11,18,19] Up to 23% of tested cats exhibited antibodies to *E cuniculi*.[16]

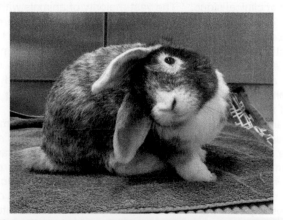

Fig. 1. Rabbit with head tilt due to encephalitozoonosis.

E cuniculi has shown zoonotic potential especially in immunocompromised humans where human immunodeficiency virus (HIV) infection has progressed to AIDS.[20] Data from the 1990s showed that strain I was most commonly found in humans in Europe, whereas the strain III isolate was more commonly identified in the Americas.[16] These varying preferences for different animals species may have reflected the popularity of rabbits and dogs as domestic pets in Europe and the Western hemisphere, respectively. Long-term shedding of spores by asymptomatic dogs has been documented, further supporting zoonotic potential.[21] Implementation of combination antiretroviral therapy (cART) to curtail HIV replication and restore immune status in HIV-infected individuals has drastically reduced the occurrence of opportunistic infections, including those due to microsporidia.[22] In developing countries where cART is not always accessible, microsporidiosis continues to be problematic. Among non-HIV-infected but immune-suppressed individuals, infections with microsporidia, although not E cuniculi specifically, have been predominately reported in organ transplant recipients and patients with malignant disease. Clinical syndromes associated with disseminated Encephalitozoon microsporidiosis in humans include encephalitis, keratoconjunctivitis, sinusitis, pneumonia, myositis, peritonitis, nephritis, and hepatitis.[22]

CLINICAL SIGNS

In principle, clinical disorders of rabbits with E cuniculi infection may include neurologic signs, renal insufficiency, as well as ocular disorders in terms of phacoclastic uveitis. However, neurologic signs have predominantly been reported.[23–25] Each of the clinical forms typically occurs individually; however, various manifestations have been documented in combination.[23–25]

Neurologic Manifestation

Most rabbits with neurologic signs show vestibular dysfunction only.[24–26] Commonly, vestibular signs have a sudden onset and can include head tilt, ataxia, nystagmus, circling movements, and rotation along the body length axis. Sometimes subtle evidence of swaying at rest or slight ataxia may be the only indication of vestibular dysfunction in rabbits with encephalitozoonosis. Vestibular signs are often observed after a stressful event in the rabbit's life. According to one study, 60% of pet rabbits with vestibular dysfunction attributable to naturally acquired encephalitozoonosis had experienced changes in their environment 72 hours before the onset of clinical signs.[27] The vast majority of animals with vestibular disorders do not exhibit other clinical signs, and even in cases of severe head tilt, food intake is still present.[25] According to one study, the degree of head tilt may serve as a major prognostic parameter in rabbits, with animals demonstrating frequent rolling and lateral recumbency having a poorer prognosis.[25] In this respect, it was recognized that a prolonged period of immobilization associated with vestibular disease may limit the recovery of the rabbit.[28] Commonly, rolling is exacerbated by handling or if the rabbit is frightened.

Neurologic examination in rabbits is carried out in a comparable manner to that in dogs and cats, keeping in mind that rabbits can be very nervous, and as prey species, may mask signs of clinical illness. The neurologic examination may be especially challenging in anxious rabbits with vestibular disease. Based on observations of spontaneous or induced sensory or motor functions, the neurologic examination is used to anatomically localize the lesion and aids in the formation of a differential diagnosis and diagnostic plan. Apart from encephalitozoonosis, otitis interna represents the main differential diagnosis in rabbits with vestibular dysfunction.[29] Therefore, veterinarians are faced with the difficulty of differentiating between peripheral vestibular dysfunction due to otitis interna and an *E cuniculi* infection causing central vestibular dysfunction. In principle, compared with a peripheral vestibular dysfunction, signs of central vestibular disorders may additionally include mentation change, cranial nerve deficits as well as postural reaction deficits. Differentiation between central and peripheral vestibular dysfunction via neurologic examination may not be possible in many cases because central vestibular disorders related to *E cuniculi* typically mimic the clinical signs of peripheral dysfunction alone.[25,26] In some cases, evidence of upper respiratory tract infection or facial nerve lesions may be more helpful in differentiating otitis interna from encephalitozoonosis. Radiography or computerized tomography is often needed to definitively differentiate the 2 diseases.

Other neurologic signs that are reported in association with encephalitozoonosis include seizures, paresis, swaying or nodding at rest, as well as behavioral changes. However, epileptic disorders might be the exception, and severe rolling may be misinterpreted as seizure activity by animal owners. A certain number of cases in which paresis or paralysis resulting from spinal cord disease were ascribed to encephalitozoonosis alone may in fact have been falsely attributed to *E cuniculi*.[25,30]

Phacoclastic Uveitis

Typical ocular lesions associated with encephalitozoonosis are widely known under the term of phacoclastic uveitis and include cataract, the development of white intraocular masses, and uveitis that can usually be detected close to the anterior lens capsule.[31–33] Most often, rabbits with phacoclastic uveitis are young individuals with unilateral ocular alterations. However, bilateral lesions, more typically found in cats, have been occasionally documented in rabbits.[11,34,35] Rabbits with ocular lesions related to encephalitozoonosis commonly do not exhibit other clinical abnormal findings. Above that, the visual impairment caused by existence of cataracts usually does not have an influence on the rabbit's quality of life (**Fig. 2**).[23,32,35]

Clinical Signs Compatible with Chronic Interstitial Nephritis

According to several studies, most rabbits with *E cuniculi*–associated kidney disease show nonspecific signs, such as polydipsia, polyuria, inappetence, weight loss, lethargy, or dehydration (**Fig. 3**).[23–25] Diagnosis is often made by the determination of urea and creatinine, and in some cases renal disease was an incidental finding detected when blood analysis was performed in middle-aged to older animals.

DIAGNOSTIC WORKUP
Serologic Testing for Specific Immunoglobulin G and Immunoglobulin M Antibodies Against Encephalitozoon cuniculi

To date, in vivo diagnosis of encephalitozoonosis in rabbits continues to be problematic because of a considerable number of rabbits having a chronic asymptomatic infection.[23,35] Therefore, ante mortem diagnosis of the neurologic form is commonly obtained by applying a combination of physical examination (including neurologic examination) and serology and by ruling out relevant differential diagnoses, such as otitis interna, purulent meningoencephalitis, trauma, and cerebral tumors.

Serology may be considered a reliable diagnostic tool for the confirmation of *E cuniculi* infections because a good correlation has been demonstrated between serologic testing and histopathology.[7,36–41] Several assays for the determination of immunoglobulin G (IgG) antibodies against *E cuniculi* such as IFAT (indirect fluorescence antibody test), enzyme-linked immunosorbent assay (ELISA), and CIA (Carbon immunoassay) are available, and it has been shown that they all correlate

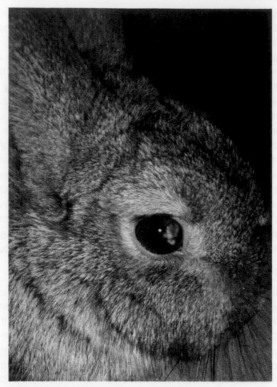

Fig. 2. Rabbit with phacoclastic uveitis associated with Encephalitozoon cuniculi infection.

well with each other.[36,42,43] However, because of the large number of asymptomatic seropositive rabbits, it must be kept in mind that the presence of antibodies may only confirm serologic evidence of pathogen exposure, and a positive serologic status is supportive for, but does not confirm *E cuniculi* as the cause of the present clinical signs.[24,25]

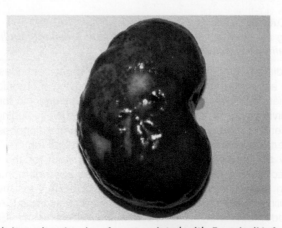

Fig. 3. Kidney with irregular pitted surface associated with *E cuniculi* infection.

Although a high correlation was demonstrated between antibody titer levels and severity of histopathologic lesions in the brain, only one study demonstrated a 1.7 higher antibody titer in animals with suspected encephalitozoonosis compared with nonsuspect rabbits.[40,43] Levels of antibody titers between rabbits with confirmed encephalitozoonosis in general do not differ significantly in comparison with titers in latent infected animals; therefore, the level of IgG antibody titers in general are unreliable for diagnostic purposes of encephalitozoonosis in rabbits.[25] However, recently, an in-house quantitative immunoblot for testing anti–*E cuniculi* antibodies in serum has been developed. This serology assay showed high diagnostic performance for *E cuniculi* infection in rabbits, with a high sensitivity for IgG and IgM detection, and almost 100% specificity for IgG and IgM, respectively.[44] This test provided a more accurate analysis of the humoral response than with conventional ELISA testing.

In contrast to seropositive results, a negative IgG antibody titer may be of diagnostic significance because of the epidemiologic characteristics of the pathogen. Seroconversion develops within approximately 3 weeks after infection and may be detected several weeks before histopathologic lesions are identified or organisms are demonstrated in tissues or body excretions.[7,37] Therefore, a negative antibody titer rules out *E cuniculi* as the cause of current disease signs.

Studies have been conducted to assess the value of specific IgM antibodies against *E cuniculi* as a diagnostic tool for the confirmation of infections in rabbits.[37,45] It was shown that specific IgM antibodies appear to be an appropriate diagnostic tool for the determination of early stages of infection, because IgM antibodies were shown to decline to zero by day 35 after an infection.[37] However, the determination of specific IgM antibodies alone is not reliable for definitive diagnosis of the disease, because the presence of the pathogen and *E cuniculi*–associated tissue alterations in predilection sites (a prerequisite for development of clinical signs) are detected not before several weeks after seroconversion has occurred.[7,37] Moreover, IgM-specific antibody titers have been demonstrated in latently infected rabbits, underlining that further investigations need to be carried out in order to evaluate the value of IgM-specific antibodies as an appropriate tool for the diagnostic workup of rabbits with suspected encephalitozoonosis.[45] The concurrent determination of both IgM and IgG may give evidence of the infection status (acute, reactivated infection, reinfection) and may therefore be helpful for in vivo diagnosis of encephalitozoonosis, but further research is needed before firm statements associating antibody titers with clinical disease can be made.

IgG antibodies against the organism have been identified in the urine samples of rabbits with confirmed infection.[46] However, results pointed out that antibodies against spore wall or polar tube of *E cuniculi* were only detected in animals with a strong seroreactivity. Further investigations are recommended about the suitability of urine as a noninvasive sample matrix for this purpose.

Polymerase Chain Reaction

Polymerase chain reaction (PCR) has long been established as the standard molecular technique for the detection of microsporidia in human medicine.[47] Several studies have been carried out to evaluate the diagnostic value of PCR for in vivo diagnosis of *E cuniculi* infections in rabbits.[26,48] PCR of liquefied lens material can be recommended as an appropriate diagnostic tool for diagnosis of phacoclastic uveitis in the living animal.[25,48] In urine samples, the value of PCR detection of *E cuniculi* organisms has been called into questions for in vivo diagnosis of the disease, because of the intermittent excretion of spores in rabbits with both clinical and asymptomatic infection.[7,25,26,37,48] PCR of cerebral spinal fluid (CSF) has been shown to be unreliable as a diagnostic tool for rabbits with neurologic signs attributable to encephalito-zoonosis based on the very low sensitivity.[26,48]

Other Diagnostic Methods for Exclusion of Relevant Differential Diagnoses

Currently, protein electrophoresis alone appears to be unreliable in the diagnostic workup of rabbits with suspected encephalitozoonosis, as changes in protein concentrations of rabbits with or without a suspicion of encephalitozoonosis did not differ significantly.[43] Although elevated C-reactive protein concentrations were detected in rabbits with E cuniculi infection, determination of C-reactive protein alone does not significantly aid in the in vivo diagnosis of encephalitozoonosis because acute phase proteins are nonspecific. However, combined determination of C-reactive protein and specific IgM and IgG antibody titers against E cuniculi may be useful in supplying a higher specificity.[49,50]

The determination of IgG antibodies against Toxoplasma gondii could theoretically be helpful in the diagnosis of rabbits with neurologic disorders. However, based on the low seroprevalence of toxoplasmosis in different rabbit populations and because of the fact that T gondii infections in rabbits are usually asymptomatic, it can only be recommended in exceptional cases.[25,51–54]

CSF analysis has been frequently applied in experimental rabbits; however, few studies have been carried out to determine its usefulness as a diagnostic tool in pet rabbits with neurologic signs. One investigation demonstrated that CSF of rabbits with a tentative diagnosis of encephalitozoonosis was characterized by a lymphomo-nocytic pleocytosis and higher protein concentrations compared with healthy rabbits.[26] Because of potential risks associated with collection and because of nonspecific alterations of CSF that may be attributed to other pathogens (eg, viruses, protozoa) or immune-mediated inflammatory diseases of the cerebrum, at this time, CSF analysis is considered an inappropriate diagnostic method for in vivo diagnosis of encephalitozoonosis.[55,56]

TREATMENT OF RABBITS WITH VESTIBULAR DYSFUNCTION

Historically, a guarded prognosis was given to rabbits with neurologic signs related to encephalitozoonosis. However, several clinical studies have been carried out to evaluate the efficacy of various drug therapies in rabbits showing vestibular dysfunction related to encephalitozoonosis with results giving a more favorable outcome.[23–25,27] In these studies, therapeutic protocols were mainly based on several fundamental principles:

- The in vitro susceptibility of microsporidial organisms to various pharmaceuticals.
- The efficacy of drugs in the treatment of human microsporidiosis in immunocompromised humans with AIDS.
- The treatment of (granulomatous) meningoencephalitis.

Although all these studies reported a recovery rate of more than 50% in rabbits with neurologic signs, it must be kept in mind that several different treatment protocols were used and studies were not controlled. In fact, few controlled studies regarding the treatment of encephalitozoonosis have been performed in the living rabbit, and in the absence of well-controlled, performed and documented scientific studies, much of current recommendations for the treatment of clinical encephalitozoonosis have been adopted based on anecdotal reports. The fact that a certain number of symptomatic rabbits may improve spontaneously without any therapy makes it even more difficult to assess the most appropriate treatment protocols.[57,58] Beyond that, response to therapy varies, and "successful treatment" has largely depended on demonstrating a resolution of clinical signs at a certain point in time after medical intervention.

To date, no uniform nor recognized treatment protocol has been established in rabbits; the authors offer a critical discussion of the principles of treatment of vestibular dysfunction associated with encephalitozoonosis.

Inhibition of Spore Proliferation

A variety of drugs have been assessed concerning the in vitro efficacy against microsporidian organisms. Certain antimicrobial substances (eg, fumagillin, sparfloxacin, oxytetracycline) and in particular the benzimidazoles (eg, albendazole, fenbendazole, oxibendazole) have been found to be effective against *E cuniculi* in a variety of studies or clinical reports.[6,59–61] Antibiotic treatment is no longer recommended in cases when otitis media/interna has been ruled out. Albendazole was identified in the mid 1990s as a successful treatment of opportunistic microsporidian infections in immunosuppressed humans during the early years of the AIDS pandemic.[62] Thereafter, the therapeutic use of albendazole was extrapolated from humans to rabbits. Since then, albendazole has been identified to be embryotoxic and teratogenic in both rats and rabbits.[63] Fenbendazole, another benzimidazole, has been shown to both prevent and treat naturally acquired as well as experimentally induced *E cuniculi* infections in rabbits using a once-daily dosage of 20 mg/kg body weight that was administered orally over a period of 28 days.[64] As a result, fenbendazole found its way into pharmaceutical formularies as a commonly used parasitostatic treatment in rabbits with encephalitozoonosis. However, despite the elimination of spores from the CNS in the Suter study, clinical signs are not always reversible in a certain number of rabbits with neurologic encephalitozoonosis. An explanation for the poor therapeutic clinical response seen in some rabbits with neurologic disorders might be due to the fact that microsporum associated the granulomatous inflammatory tissue alterations within the brain remain despite a successful reduction in the number of infectious spores. To add to the confusion of what determines successful treatment is the fact that *E cuniculi* infections typically follow a chronic course whereby the manifestation of clinical signs vary and the time from infection until clinical encephalitozoonosis may be months to years and almost always occurs long after initial infection and when only a low number of organisms are present within affected tissues.[40] Consistent with this, a recent study showed that oral administration of fenbendazole before experimental infection was effective to some extent in protection of rabbits against infection with *E cuniculi*.[65] This same study failed to observe significant effects on clinical signs when administered as a treatment.[65] Even though the true efficacy of antiparasitic treatment is often called into question based on the lack of completeness of current studies, the low numbers of spores present in tissues, and the severe inflammatory alterations that result from infection, fenbendazole still remains an essential part of the treatment regimen in most rabbits with neurologic disorders due to of encephalitozoonosis. Adverse reactions in terms of crypt necrosis of small intestine or bone marrow hypoplasia/aplasia have been reported with the use of benzimidazoles in rabbits, and as a result, practitioners should strictly adhere to recommended dosages and treatment intervals when using benzimidazole derivatives and consider monitoring complete blood counts during treatment.[64,66]

Anti-Inflammatory Therapy

The clinical disorders associated with *E cuniculi* may not be associated with the presence of the organism itself, but rather with the inflammatory lesions that develop when cells rupture and spores are released into surrounding tissues.[67] It is known that this inflammatory reaction tends to be granulomatous in nature and may persist after the organism is no longer present.[40] As a result, the use of glucocorticoids has anecdotally been advised for the treatment of rabbits with neurologic disorders because of encephalitozoonosis. However, a recently conducted investigation did not support the use of dexamethasone as an effective treatment modality for rabbits with neurologic disorders attributable to encephalitozoonosis.[68] The use of prednisolone or dexamethasone is controversial primarily because of their potential immunosuppressive effects.[58,69] As well, glucocorticoids are known to influence the cell-mediated immune response, the main defense mechanism against the pathogen. The usefulness of systemic anti-inflammatory treatment is also called into question because of the fact that tissue damage that occurs during the course of encephalitozoonosis is commonly irreversible. It has been shown that severe histologic lesions of the predilection sites (brain and kidney) attributable to *E cuniculi* are not necessarily associated with clinical disease and that histopathologic examination of the CNS revealed no significant differences in regard to the severity and distribution of inflammatory brain changes in rabbits with both latent and clinical *E cuniculi* infection, again calling into question the usefulness of corticosteroid anti-inflammatories in the treatment of encephalitozoonosis.[40] The use of nonsteroidal anti-inflammatory drugs (NSAIDs) may well also be questionable for similar reasons; to the authors' knowledge, no studies exist on the use of NSAIDs for therapeutic treatment of encephalitozoonosis in rabbits.

Supportive Care

The vestibular signs associated with encephalitozoonosis tend not to diminish the appetite in rabbits and most continue to eat well even if they cannot maintain an upright position. Therefore, in contrast to dogs and cats, prevention of nausea secondary to vestibular disorders with the use of prokinetics, antiemetics, or drugs designed to control dizziness (metoclopramide, prochloroperazine, meclizine) is usually not recommended.[25] Assist feeding is used as needed but often not indicated. In cases of severe vestibular dysfunction, it must be assured that immobilized rabbits are caged in a quiet and stress-free environment and can reach the offered food.[69] In order to prevent injury, padded cages should be provided for rabbits that are severely rolling.[58,69] Alternatively, rabbits with severe vestibular signs may benefit from treatment with benzodiazepines (diazepam, midazolam) that relax the patient and thus minimize the neurologic signs associated with acute vestibular dysfunction.[25,58]

Physiotherapy: Therapeutic Exercise

Recently, it has been recognized that physical therapy has an important impact on the improvement of clinical disease in rabbits with vestibular dysfunction.[25,58] Encouraging activity early in the course of disease and adding in therapeutic exercise may even represent the most important part of therapy in rabbits with vestibular dysfunction when it is designed to appropriately challenge the nervous system deficits and strengthen the musculoskeletal system, allowing for an earlier return to more normal independent patient function.[58] Therapeutic exercise should be performed on a slip-resistant surface and may include different training techniques that may help to compensate for vestibular deficits. Physical exercises vary depending on the severity of vestibular deficits, such as lateral recumbent position, rolling, or circling. In this sense, exercises may comprise simple assistance to maintain an upright position, support to minimize grade of head tilt, and help the animal in making straight forward movements. In many cases, it has proved to be sufficient to provide an opportunity for free run under strict supervision of a person that can provide support immediately if the rabbit rotates. The possibility for free run on a slip-resistant surface should be offered several times a day for 10 to 30 minutes dependent on the severity of disease signs.

Preferably, rabbits with severe vestibular disorders should be hospitalized as even experienced rabbit owners are often overstrained with 24-hour care of those patients.

In contrast, a period of immobilization following an acute onset of vestibular dysfunction not only slows recovery but also may actually impair the recovery of vestibular function.[28,58] Although most rabbits improve with physiotherapy in the form of gradually increased exercise, residual deficits (mostly minor head tilt) may persist in a certain number of treated rabbits.

REFERENCES

1. Didier ES, Weiss LM. Microsporidiosis: current status. Curr Opin Infect Dis 2006; 19(5):485–92.
2. Katinka MD, Duprat S, Cornillot E, et al. Genome sequence and gene compaction of the eukaryote parasite Encephalitozoon cuniculi. Nature 2001;414:450–3.
3. Bohn W, Böttcher K, Gross U. The parasitophorous vacuole of Encephalitozoon cuniculi: Biogenesis characteristics of the host cell-pathogen interface. Int J Med Microbiol 2011;301:395–9.
4. Franzen C, Muller A, Hartmann P, et al. Cell invasion and intracellular fate of Encephalitozoon cuniculi (Microsporidia). Parasitology 2005;130:285–92.
5. Hunt C. Radiographic interpretation of the vertebral column. In: Harcourt-Brown F, Chitty J, editors. BSAVA manual of rabbit surgery, dentistry and imaging. Gloucester (United Kingdom): BSAVA Publications; 2013. p. 76–83.
6. Franssen FF, Lumeij JT, van Knapen F. Susceptibility of Encephalitozoon cuniculi to several drugs in vitro. Antimicrob Agents Chemother 1995;39:1265–8.
7. Cox JC, Gallichio HA. Serological and histological studies on adult rabbits with recent, naturally acquired encephalitozoonosis. Res Vet Sci 1978;24:260–1.
8. Lyngset A. A survey of serum antibodies to Encephalitozoon cuniculi in breeding rabbits and their young. Lab Anim Sci 1980;30:558–61.
9. Didier ES, Didier PJ, Snowden KF, et al. Microspordiosis in mammals. Microbes Infect 2000;2:709–12.
10. Talabani H, Sarfati C, Pillebout E, et al. Disseminated infection with a new genovar of Encephalitozoon cuniculi in a renal transplant recipient. J Clin Microbiol 2010; 48(7):2651–3.
11. Benz P, Maaß G, Csokai J, et al. Detection of Encephalitozoon cuniculi in the feline cataractous lens. Vet Ophthalmol 2011;14:37–47.
12. Illanes OG, Tiffani-Castiglioni E, Edwards JF, et al. Spontaneous encephalitozoonosis in an experimental group of guinea pigs. J Vet Diagn Invest 1993;5:649–51.
13. Boot R, Van Knapen F, Kruijt BC, et al. Serological evidence for Encephalitozoon cuniculi infection (nosemiasis) in gnotobiotic guinea pigs. Lab Anim 1988;22: 337–42.
14. Majeeb SK, Zubaidy AJ. Histopathological lesions associated with Encephalitozoon cuniculi (nosematosis) infection in a colony of Wistar rats. Lab Anim 1982; 16:244–7.
15. Muller-Doblies UU, Herzog K, Tanner I, et al. First isolation and characterization of Encephalitozoon cuniculi from a free-ranging rat (Rattus norvegicus). Vet Parasitol 2002;107(4):279–85.

16. Jordan CN. Encephalitozoon cuniculi: diagnostic test and methods of inactivation. [Author thesis]. Blacksburg (VA): Faculty of the Virginia Polytechnic Institute and State University; 2005. p. 23.

17. Snowden KF, Lewis BC, Hoffman J, et al. Encephalitozoon cuniculi infections in dogs: a case series. J Am Anim Hosp Assoc 2009;45(5):225–31.

18. Csokai J, Fuchs-Baumgartinger A, Maas G, et al. Detection of Encephalitozoon cuniculi-infection (strain II) by PCR in a cat with anterior uveitis. Wien Tierarztl Monatsschr 2010;97:210–5.

19. Scurrell EJ, Holding E, Hopper J, et al. Bilateral lenticular Encephalitozoon cuniculi infection in a snow leopard (Panthera uncia). Vet Ophthalmol 2015; 18(Supplement 1):143–7.

20. Didier ES, Maddry JA, Brindley PJ, et al. Therapeutic strategies for human microsporidia infections. Expert Rev Anti Infect Ther 2005;3:419–34.

21. Snowden K, Logan K, Didier ES. Encephalitozoon cuniculi strain III is a cause of Encephalitozoonosis in both humans and dogs. J Infect Dis 1999;180:2086–8.

22. Didier ES, Weiss LM. Microsporidiosis: not just in AIDS patients. Curr Opin Infect Dis 2011;24(5):490–5.

23. Ewringmann A, Göbel T. Untersuchungen zur Klinik und Therapie der Enzephalitozoonose beim Heimtierkaninchen. Kleintierprax 1999;44:357–72.

24. Harcourt-Brown FM, Holloway HK. Encephalitozoon cuniculi in pet rabbits. Vet Rec 2003;152:427–31.

25. Künzel F, Gruber A, Tichy A, et al. Clinical symptoms and diagnosis of encephalitozoonosis in pet rabbits. Vet Parasitol 2008;151:115–24.

26. Jass A, Matiasek K, Henke J, et al. Analysis of cerebrospinal fluid in healthy rabbits and rabbits with clinically suspected encephalitozoonosis. Vet Rec 2008;162: 618–22.

27. Meyer-Breckwoldt A. Epidemiologische und klinische Untersuchungen zur Encephalitozoonose beim Zwergkaninchen [Dissertation]. Hannover (Germany): Veterinary University; 1996.

28. Thomas WB. Vestibular dysfunction. Vet Clin North Am Small Anim Pract 2000;30: 227–49.

29. Gruber A, Pakozdy A, Weissenböck H, et al. A retrospective study of neurological disease in 118 rabbits. J Comp Pathol 2009;14:31–7.

30. Künzel F, Joachim A. Encephalitozoonosis in rabbits. Parasitol Res 2010;106: 299–309.

31. Grahn B, Wolfer J, Keller Ch. Diagnostic ophthalmology. Can Vet J 1991;32: 372–3.

32. Fechle LM, Sigler RL. Phacoemulsification for the management of Encephalitozoonon cuniculi-induced phacoclastic uveitis in a rabbit. Vet Ophthalmol 2002; 5:211–5.

33. Giordano C, Weigt A, Vercelli A, et al. Immunohistochemical identification of Encephalitozoon cuniculi in phacoclastic uveitis in four rabbits. Vet Ophthalmol 2005;8:271–5.

34. Ashton N, Cook C, Clegg F. Encephalitozoonosis (nosematosis) causing bilateral cataract in a rabbit. Br J Ophthalmol 1976;60:618–31.

35. Harcourt-Brown FM. Encephalitozoon cuniculi infection in rabbits. Semin Avian Exot Pet Med 2004;13:86–93.

36. Waller T. The India-ink immunoreaction: a method for the rapid diagnosis of encephalitozoonosis. Lab Anim 1977;11:93–7.

37. Cox JC, Hamilton RC, Attwood HD. An investigation of the route and progression of Encephalitozoon cuniculi infection in adult rabbits. J Protozool 1979;26:260–5.

38. Scharmann W, Reblin L, Griem W. Infection of rabbits with Encephalitozoon cuniculi. Berl Munch Tierarztl Wochenschr 1986;99:20–4.
39. Eröksüz Y, Eröksüz H, Özer H, et al. A survey of Encephalitozoon cuniculi infection in rabbit colonies in Elazig, Turkey: pathomorphologic and serlogic (carbon-immunoassay test) studies. Isr J Vet Med 1999;54:73–7.
40. Csokai J, Gruber A, Künzel F, et al. Encephalitozoonosis in pet rabbits (Oryctolagus cuniculus): pathohistological findings in animals with latent infection versus clinical manifestation. Parasitol Res 2009;104:629–35.
41. Hein J, Flock U, Sauter-Louis C, et al. Encephalitozoon cuniculi in rabbits in Germany: prevalence and sensitivity of antibody testing. Vet Rec 2014;174(14):350.
42. Tee KY, Kao JP, Chiu HY, et al. Serological survey for antibodies to Encephalitozoon cuniculi in rabbits in Taiwan. Vet Parasitol 2011;83(1–2):68–71.
43. Cray C, Arcia G, Schneider R, et al. Evaluation of the usefulness of an ELISA and protein electrophoresis in the diagnosis of Encephalitozoon cuniculi infection in rabbits. Am J Vet Res 2009;70:478–82.
44. Desoubeaux G, Pantin A, Peschke R, et al. Application of Western blot analysis for the diagnosis of Encephalitozoon cuniculi infection in rabbits: example of a quantitative approach. Parasitol Res 2017;116(2):743–50.
45. Jeklova E, Jekl V, Kovarcik K, et al. Usefulness of detection of specific IgM and IgG antibodies for diagnosis of clinical encephalitozoonosis in pet rabbits. Vet Parasitol 2010;170:143–8.
46. Furuya K, Asakura T, Igarashi M, et al. Microsporidian Encephalitozoon cuniculi antibodies in rabbit urine samples. Vet Rec 2009;165(3):85–6.
47. Katzwinkel-Wladarsch S, Deplazes P, Weber R, et al. Comparison of polymerase chain reaction with light microscopy for detection of microsporidia in clinical specimens. Eur J Clin Microbiol Infect Dis 1997;16:7–10.
48. Csokai J, Joachim A, Gruber A, et al. Diagnostic markers for encephalitozoonosis in pet rabbits. Vet Parasitol 2009;163:18–26.
49. Cray C, Rodriguez M, Fernandez Y. Acute phase protein levels in rabbits with suspected Encephalitozoon cuniculi infection. J Exot Pet Med 2013;22:280–6.
50. Cray C, McKenny S, Perritt E, et al. Utility of IgM titers with IgG and C-reactive protein quantitation in the diagnosis of suspected Encephalitozoon cuniculi infection in rabbits. J Exot Ped Med 2015;24:356–60.
51. Leland MM, Hubbard GV, Dubey JP. Clinical toxoplasmosis in domestic rabbits. Lab Anim Sci 1992;42:318–9.
52. Neumayerová H, Juránková J, Jeklová E, et al. Seroprevalence of Toxoplasma gondii and Encephalitozoon cuniculi in rabbits from different farming systems. Vet Parasitol 2014;204(3–4):184–90.
53. Salman D, Oohashi E, Mohamed AE, et al. Seroprevalences of Toxoplasma gondii and Neospora caninum in pet rabbits in Japan. J Vet Med Sci 2014;76(6):855–62.
54. Fisher PG, Carpenter JW. Neurologic and musculoskeletal disease. In: Quesenberry KE, Carpenter JW, editors. Ferrets, rabbits and rodents: clinical medicine and surgery. 3rd edition. St Louis (MO): Saunders Elsevier; 2012. p. 245–56.
55. Ludwig H, Köster V, Pauli G, et al. The cerebrospinal fluid of rabbits infected with Borna disease virus. Arch Virol 1977;55:209–23.
56. Summers BA, Cummings JF, Lahunta A. Veterinary neuropathology. St Louis (MO): Mosby; 1999.
57. Valencakova A, Balent P, Petrovova E, et al. Encephalitozoonosis in household pet Nederland Dwarf rabbits (Oryctolagus cuniculus). Vet Parasitol 2008;153(3–4):265–9.

58. Harcourt-Brown FM. Infectious diseases of domestic rabbits. In: Harcourt-Brown FM, editor. Textbook of rabbit medicine. Oxford: Butterworth-Heinemann; 2002. p. 361–85.
59. Waller T. Sensitivity of Encephalitozoon cuniculi to various temperatures, disinfectants and drugs. Lab Anim 1979;13:227–30.
60. Shadduck JA. Effect of fumagillin on in vitro multiplication of Encephalitozoon cuniculi. J Protozool 1980;27(2):202–8.
61. Beauvais B, Sarfati C, Challier S, et al. In vitro model to assess effect of antimicrobial agents on Encephalitozoon cuniculi. Antimicrob Agents Chemother 1994; 38(10):2440–8.
62. De Groote MA, Visvesvara G, Wilson ML, et al. Polymerase chain reaction and culture confirmation of disseminated Encephalitozoon cuniculi in a patient with AIDS: successful therapy with albendazole. J Infect Dis 1995;171:1375–8.
63. Kotler DP, Orenstein JM. Clinical syndromes associated with microsporidiosis. Adv Parasitol 1998;40:321–49.
64. Suter C, Müller-Doblies UU, Hatt JM, et al. Prevention and treatment of Encephalitozoon cuniculi infection in rabbits with fenbendazole. Vet Rec 2001;148:478–80.
65. Abu-Akkada SS, Oda SS. Prevention and treatment of Encephalitozoon cuniculi infection in immunosuppressed rabbits with fenbendazole. Iran J Vet Res 2016; 17(2):98–105.
66. Graham JE, Garner MM, Reavill DR. Benzimidazole toxicosis in rabbits: 13 cases (2003-2011). J Educ Perioper Med 2014;23(2):188–95.
67. Feaga WP. Wry neck in rabbits. J Am Vet Med Assoc 1997;210:480.
68. Sieg J, Hein J, Jass A, et al. Clinical evaluation of therapeutic success in rabbits with suspected encephalitozoonosis. Vet Parasitol 2012;187:328–32.
69. Keeble E. Encephalitozoonosis in rabbits–what we do and don't know. In Pract 2011;33:426–35.

Analgesics in Small Mammals

Paul Flecknell, MA, VetMB, PhD, DECLAM, DLAS, DECVAA, FRSB[a,b,]*

KEYWORDS

- Pain assessment • Analgesia • Analgesics • Rodents • Rabbits • Rat • Mouse
- Guinea pig

KEY POINTS

- Effective use of analgesics in small mammals requires pain intensity to be assessed. After assessing the intensity of pain, an analgesic regimen can be formulated and administered and its efficacy confirmed by repeated pain assessment.
- Pain assessment tools are still in an early stage of development, but assessment of specific behaviors and use of grimace scales to assess facial expression can be used in many species.
- Analgesic dosage recommendations are based largely on clinical experience, but information is gradually accumulating based on objective assessment of efficacy in clinically relevant settings.

INTRODUCTION

Managing pain effectively in any species is challenging, but small mammals present some particular problems. This clinical review focuses on pain assessment and pain alleviation in rats, mice, guinea pigs, and rabbits, because there is a reasonable evidence base in these species on which to base clinical decisions. Suggestions are made as to how to extrapolate information to other species, such as gerbils, hamsters, degus, and chinchillas.

Although the underlying mechanisms of nociception and pain are similar in all mammals that present for veterinary treatment, detecting pain can be particularly difficult in rodents and rabbits. But if the presence of pain cannot be recognized and its intensity assessed, then analgesics cannot be used effectively. If pain fails to be detected, it may be considered there is no need to administer analgesics. If pain is suspected to be present but how much pain an animal is experiencing cannot be assessed, then the analgesic protocol cannot be adjusted to suit the need of each individual. If

Disclosure Statement: The author has no conflicts of interest or competing interests.
[a] Comparative Biology Centre, Medical School, Newcastle University, Framlington Place, Newcastle NE24RU, UK; [b] Flaire Consultants
* Corresponding author.
E-mail address: Paul.flecknell@ncl.ac.uk

an analgesic is given, the reduction in pain must be able to be assessed to determine that the drug selected and the dose rate used have been effective in that individual animal.

Pain assessment in dogs and cats is not always straightforward, but most veterinary surgeons and veterinary technicians are familiar with the normal behavior of these species. The normal behavior and general appearance of small rodents, ferrets, and rabbits are often less well appreciated, so that signs associated with pain may be overlooked. In addition, several species of small mammals are nocturnal and may not be active when observed during normal working hours. They may also remain immobile in the presence of an observer if they perceive them as a threat. This can be a particular problem with rabbits and guinea pigs. Although it is not always easy to use behavior and changes in appearance to assess pain, it is important to overcome these difficulties so that pain can be prevented or controlled effectively in these small animals.

GENERAL SIGNS OF PAIN

As with dogs and cats, an initial assessment of a small mammal should be made without disturbing it. The animal's appearance and posture may be abnormal and it may appear hunched. Its coat may be unkempt and ruffled because of a lack of grooming and the presence of piloerection. Rats may have a blackish discharge around their eyes and nose, due to a build-up of secretions from their harderian glands. This build-up of material is a nonspecific response to ill health, pain, and other stress, but in the postoperative period it is a useful indicator that the animal could be in pain. While an animal is observed, it may demonstrate normal inquisitive behavior and explore its environment, but, as discussed previously, if it remains motionless this may be because it feels threatened rather than because it is in pain. If an animal has positioned itself in the back of its cage or pen or has hidden in bedding, this can also be a sign of fear but may also be due to pain.

Observing spontaneous behavior in a veterinary practice setting can be challenging—the smells, sounds, and sight of other patients, who may be predators of small mammals, may result in suppression of all behavior. If an area can be found that is free from both sounds and odors of predators, this helps assessment, and it is also now simple to set up remote observation of animals using a webcam or tethered camera system. Using a security-style camera with infrared sensitivity also allows observation during the dark phase of an animal's photoperiod, when many small mammals should be very active. Aside from allowing more reliable observations to be made, a quiet area away from predators reduces the stress associated with hospitalization and reduces the risk of stress-related problems, such as gastrointestinal disorders in rabbits and guinea pigs.

After observing an animal in as undisturbed state as possible, it should be approached and examined. When encouraged to move, the animal may have an abnormal gait or posture and may show uncharacteristic signs of aggression. Rats, mice, and gerbils usually rear when investigating what has disturbed them and the absence of this behavior may be due to pain. When handled, rather than attempting to evade capture, animals in pain may be apathetic or, as discussed previously, may be aggressive and bite the handler. When examining an animal, it may respond to manipulation or palpation of a painful area by vocalizing or trying to bite. Some mammals, such as guinea pigs, also vocalize loudly when not in pain and may respond to any manipulation by tensing their muscles and remaining immobile. Similar unresponsiveness can also be seen in rabbits. When examining small mammals, such as mice, hamsters, and gerbils, use of a clear acrylic handling tube allows good observation, without the need for firm physical restraint (**Fig. 1**). This method of handling has also been shown to reduce stress and anxiety.[1,2]

SPECIFIC SIGNS OF PAIN

The changes, discussed previously, are nonspecific signs of pain. They can also occur as a result of general ill health but are nevertheless useful when other examinations suggest pain could be present, for example, due to otitis, dental disease, or arthritis. They can also be helpful when assessing animals after surgical procedures when some pain is inevitable unless particularly effective pain management strategies have been implemented.

The management of pain in dogs and cats has been greatly improved by the development of validated pain scales, incorporating behavioral changes that are reliable indicators of pain. In small mammals and rabbits, such scales are in a much earlier stage of development. Nevertheless, pain that has a visceral component, for example, after abdominal surgery or after orchidectomy, often produces some characteristic behaviors in rats, mice, rabbits, and guinea pigs.[3–7] Given the shared characteristics of these behaviors, it is probable that similar behaviors are also of value in assessing pain in other, less familiar species.

Rats, mice, rabbits, and guinea pigs may show contraction of the abdominal muscles, producing a hollowed-out appearance to the flanks (**Figs. 2–4**). Rats, mice, and rabbits may also press their abdomen to the ground (**Fig. 5**). Rats may arch their backs (**Fig. 6**) and rats, mice, and rabbits may stagger when performing normal behaviors. If a rat or mouse is in moderate or severe pain, these behaviors are seen frequently, for example, 4 to 5 abnormal behaviors in a 5-minute to 10-minute period. Rabbits show a similar frequency but may only do so if observed remotely. Even well-socialized rabbits, with a familiar observer, may reduce the incidence of these behaviors. Guinea pigs are even less demonstrative, and a prolonged period of observation, using remote monitoring, for 15 minutes to 30 minutes may be needed to identify these behavioral changes.[7] Achieving this in a busy veterinary practice may be impracticable, but other means of assessing pain, using facial expression (discussed later), may be more useful.

Anecdotally, rabbits with abdominal pain are said to grind their teeth, but this may not always be pain related. The author has also never observed this behavior in studies of pain related behavior in rabbits. Rabbits and all small mammals may stop eating and

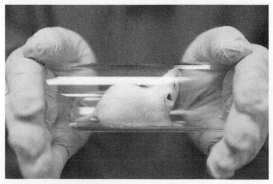

Fig. 1. Use of a handling tube to examine a mouse —the animal is encouraged to run into the tube while in its cage or transport box.

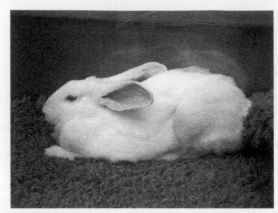

Fig. 2. Rabbit showing abdominal contraction due to pain after surgery (ovariohysterectomy) and insufficient analgesia. The animal is also showing some facial expression changes associated with pain (see **Fig. 12**).

drinking when experiencing pain. This can be difficult to detect because food is often provided as desired, but the consequent loss in body weight can easily be monitored.[8] This is one of the simplest ways of following an animal's progress after surgery or during treatment of any disease condition. A fall in food and water consumption caused by pain is a serious problem in small mammals, because failure to drink can rapidly lead to significant dehydration, and lack of food intake can predispose to the development of hypoglycemia in small mammals. In addition, in rabbits, guinea pigs, and chinchillas, disturbances in food intake can lead to the development of life-threatening gastrointestinal disturbances.

Rats and mice in pain reduce their performance of some highly motivated behaviors, such as burrowing and nest building. Measurement of these behaviors has been used to assess pain in carefully controlled studies,[9,10] and the approach could prove useful in a clinical setting. Mice in pain build less well-constructed nests and are slower to build a nest. Assessing nesting behavior before and after surgery might provide additional information as to the efficacy of analgesia. Digging behavior is less easy to assess in a home cage environment, but the methods used (filling a small bottle

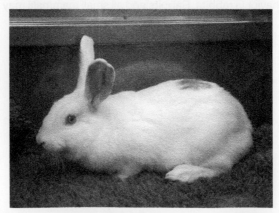

Fig. 3. Rabbit showing normal profile to the abdomen and normal posture after abdominal surgery with the provision of effective analgesia.

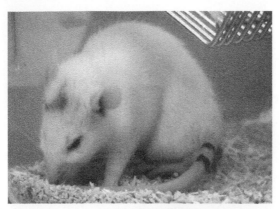

Fig. 4. Rat showing abdominal contraction and partial back arch due to postoperative abdominal pain.

with gravel or with diet pellets) is easy to implement.[11] This approach has been shown effective in detecting chronic inflammatory and neuropathic pain in rats so has the potential to be used to diagnose chronic painful conditions. Demonstrating an increase in burrowing after administration of an analgesic confirms the presence of pain and allows monitoring of analgesic efficacy.

RODENT AND RABBIT GRIMACE SCALES (PAIN FACES)

Most pet owners and many veterinarians consider they can assess the emotional state of an animal from its facial expressions. Charles Darwin considered facial expressions as indicating a range of emotions and noted that similar expressions were shared across different species and between animals and humans.[12] Applying this approach in an objective way to assess pain is a recent development.[13] After the initial demonstration that mice show characteristic pain faces that could be used to develop a mouse grimace scale (**Figs. 7** and **8**), similar scales have been developed in other species. Rats have been shown to have facial expressions characteristic of pain[14] (**Figs. 9** and **10**) as have rabbits[15] (**Figs. 11–13**). Grimace scales have also been developed in horses,[16] sheep and lambs,[17,18] and pigs,[19] and similar approaches may be applicable in a wide range of species.[20]

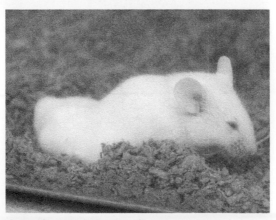

Fig. 5. Mouse showing a characteristic press due to postsurgical abdominal pain.

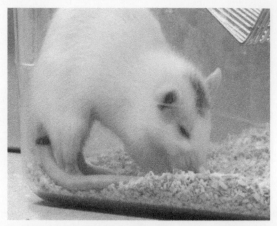

Fig. 6. Back arching caused by abdominal pain after laparotomy in the rat.

The expressions shown can be used to evaluate the degree of pain but care must be taken because other factors can also result in animals showing these facial expressions.[21] An attraction of using grimace scales is that similar changes seem to occur with different types and sources of pain and can be easily captured by both direct observations and use of video and still images. This approach is still at an early stage of development, but initial studies suggest it can be used as a cageside means of assessing pain.[22,23] Facial expression may also be less susceptible to changing as a result of the nonspecific effects of analgesics. This can be a problem when using other behavioral assessments—for example, opioids can either increase activity (in mice and gerbils) or cause sedation (in rats and rabbits). Using grimace scales in combination with the other indicators, described previously, may provide the best means of assessing pain in many species, not only small mammals.

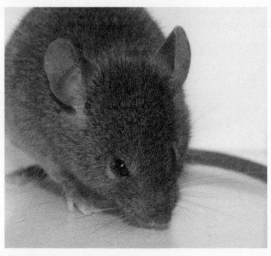

Fig. 7. Normal facial expression in the mouse.

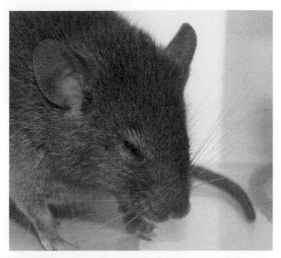

Fig. 8. Pain face in the mouse—showing nose bulging, orbital tightening, and cheek bulge.

ASSESSING PAIN IN CLINICAL PRACTICE

As experience is gained in observing the normal behavior patterns of small mammals and rabbits, changes in the frequency of normal behaviors and the occurrence of abnormal behaviors are detected with greater confidence. Although specific signs of pain, such as guarding of an injured area, may be seen, many of the signs are nonspecific and can also occur in response to nonpainful conditions. It is, therefore, important to consider the appearance of the animal in relation to its case history and other clinical findings. It is also important to appreciate that pain assessment

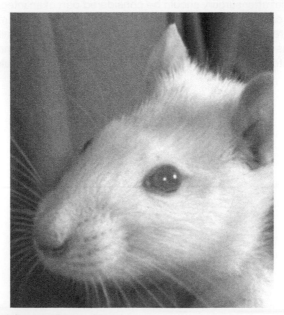

Fig. 9. Normal facial expression in the rat.

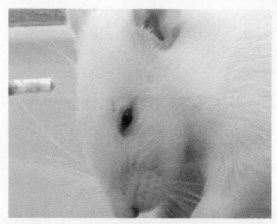

Fig. 10. Pain face in the rat—showing ear changes, orbital tightening, and clumping of whiskers.

takes time—observing specific abnormal behaviors takes 5 minutes to 10 minutes per animal to allow effective assessments. Observing general behavior and activity takes even longer. Couple this with the relative lack of familiarity veterinarians have, and it is clear that one of the best people to assess pain in a companion animal is the owner. Encouraging owners of animals to make detailed assessments, especially in combination with administration of therapy, may be a valuable adjunct to assessments in the clinic.

PAIN PREVENTION AND ALLEVIATION
Postoperative and Posttrauma Pain

Effective pain relief after surgery should be considered part of an integrated approach to perioperative care. There is extensive evidence in people that stress and anxiety increase the degree of pain experienced and increase the need for pain relief. In addition, veterinarians should be concerned to alleviate both distress and discomfort as well as pain. Postoperative pain relief is important in all small mammals, but providing

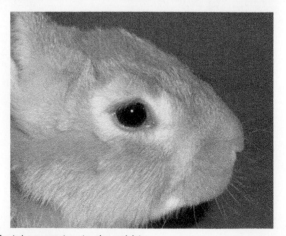

Fig. 11. Normal facial expression in the rabbit.

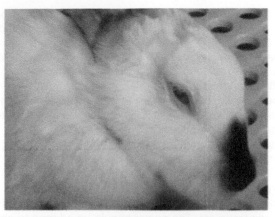

Fig. 12. Pain face in the rabbit—showing marked orbital tightening.

pain relief in rabbits and guinea pigs is especially important to ensure an uncomplicated recovery from surgery. As in other species, the most obvious means of preventing pain is by administration of analgesic drugs; however, the choice of drug and the timing of its administration should be considered carefully. It is also important not to overlook other important factors, for example, careful surgical technique with gentle handling of tissues reduces the degree of postoperative pain. Analgesic use should also be combined with nutritional and fluid and support and general nursing care. These considerations apply to all species, but in small mammals several particular issues need greater attention.[24] Small mammals are particularly susceptible to developing hypothermia during anesthesia. Most anesthetic protocols include provision of warming, but this must be continued into the postoperative period. A suitable recovery area should be established as part of the preoperative preparations, so that it can be stabilized at an appropriate temperature. Initially a temperature of approximately 35°C should be maintained and this can be lowered to 26°C to 28°C as the animal recovers consciousness. Animals should be provided with warm, comfortable bedding. A layer of synthetic fleece should be provided for the initial recovery period, but once

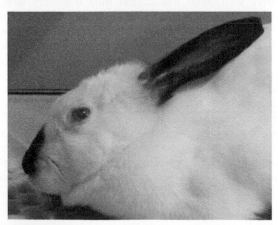

Fig. 13. Pain face in the rabbit—showing folding and flattening of the ears and orbital tightening.

the animal has regained activity it can be transferred to a cage or pen containing its normal bedding and nesting material. Rabbits and guinea pigs should be provided with good quality hay or straw. This type of bedding allows the animal to surround itself with insulating material, which provides both warmth and a sense of security. It also encourages them to eat as soon as possible, so helping prevent development of gastrointestinal disturbances.

Water should be provided, but care must be taken that this does not spill, because if the animal becomes wet it loses heat rapidly. Small rodents are usually used to using sipper bottles, as are rabbits, so this is not usually a problem, but it can present difficulties if a bowl is used for rabbits and guinea pigs. Even after uncomplicated anesthesia and surgery and with good analgesia, fluid intake may be reduced, so routine administration of warmed (37°C) subcutaneous or intraperitoneal dextrose/saline at the end of surgery is advisable.

Provided an animal has recovered well from anesthesia, it is probably best returned home to a familiar environment. The owner should be advised to observe the animal closely for the next few days, to be sure it is eating and drinking and passing feces. Establishing effective analgesia before discharging from the clinical helps ensure the animal recovers well.

Analgesic Agents

As in other species, a range of different analgesics is available, including nonsteroidal anti-inflammatory drugs (NSAIDs), opioids, and local anesthetics. Information concerning appropriate dose rates has been drawn from a variety of sources. Some species of small mammals have been used in laboratory evaluations of the safety and efficacy of analgesic agents. Extensive data of this type are available for rats and mice, but there is less information concerning rabbits, guinea pigs, hamsters, and gerbils. There are no data of this type for the less common small mammals, such as chinchillas and chipmunks. The information provided by laboratory studies is useful and provides information of safety and efficacy, in particular analgesic tests. The tests are not always directly relevant to the types of pain seen in veterinary practice, however, so dose rates need to be estimated carefully. It is also important to note that these studies were carried out in healthy laboratory animals, in controlled environmental conditions. Administration of analgesics to animals in poor health or use of analgesics concurrently with other medication may markedly alter an individual's response. Unfortunately, there are few studies of the efficacy of analgesics in clinically relevant situations. The majority of information has, therefore, been obtained from clinical experience. Dose rates are often recommended based on dose rates initially estimated by extrapolation from other species. When applied in clinical situations and found to be at least safe, these dose rates become established in textbooks and review articles,[25] even if efficacy has not been evaluated reliably. It is, therefore, important to continue to review analgesic use because recommendations change more frequently than for the more familiar companion animal species.

Fortunately, clinical experience suggests that the analgesics that are frequently used in dogs and cats can all be used safely for the control of postoperative pain in small mammals and rabbits. Although none of the agents listed in **Table 1** has manufacturer recommendations for small mammals, many are extensively used both in clinical practice and in laboratory animals.

Nonsteroidal anti-inflammatory drugs

Although it is likely that all the agents currently available for use in companion animals can be used safely in small mammals and rabbits, most published data are available

Table 1
Analgesics for use in small mammals. Suggested dose rates based on clinical experience of the author and other colleagues. None of these agents has manufacturer recommendations for use in these species. Effects vary in individual animals, and each animal should be assessed to try to determine the efficacy of the analgesic

Analgesic	Gerbil and Hamster	Guinea Pig	Mouse	Rat	Rabbit
Buprenorphine	0.1 mg/kg sc, ?6–8 hourly	0.05 mg/kg sc, 6–12 hourly	0.1 mg/kg sc, 4–8 hourly	0.05 mg/kg sc, 4–8 hourly	0.01–0.05 mg/kg sc or IV, 6–12 hourly
Butorphanol	?	2 mg/kg sc, 2 hourly	1–5 mg/kg sc, 2 hourly	2 mg/kg sc, 2 hourly	0.1–0.5 mg/kg sc or IV, 2 hourly
Carprofen	5 mg/kg sc, ? daily	4 mg/kg sc, ? daily	5 mg/kg sc, bid	5 mg/kg sc or orally, daily	1.5 mg/kg po, 4 mg/kg sc or IV
Meloxicam	?	0.5–1.0 mg/kg sc or orally, ? daily	5 mg/kg sc or orally, bid	1 mg/kg sc or orally, ? daily	0.4–0.6 mg/kg po, 0.4–0.6 mg/kg sc, ? daily
Morphine	?	2–5 mg/kg sc or IM, 4 hourly	5 mg/kg sc or IM, 4 hourly	2.5 mg/kg sc or IM, 4 hourly	2 mg/kg sc, IM, 3–4 hourly
Meperidine	?	10–20 mg/kg sc or IM, 2–3 hourly	10–20 mg/kg sc or IM, 2–3 hourly	10–20 mg/kg sc or IM, 2–3 hourly	?
Tramadol	?	?	5 mg/kg sc, IP or po	5 mg/kg sc, IP or po	?

?, insufficient data to recommend dose rates.
Abbreviations: bid, twice a day; IM, intramuscularly; IP, interperitoneal; po, per os (by mouth); sc, subcutaneous.
Data from Flecknell and Waterman-Pearson, 2000, "Pain management in animals", Flecknell, "Laboratory animal anaesthesia, 2015, clinical experience.

for meloxicam and carprofen. There seems some marked species variation in efficacy of NSAIDs, with very high dose rates required in mice (20 mg/kg) in comparison with rats (1 mg/kg) for postoperative analgesia.[26–28] Similarly in rabbits, high doses of meloxicam are needed for postoperative analgesia, and these need to be combined with local anesthesia or opioids for effective pain relief,[6,29,30] illustrating the care needed when extrapolating between species, without the means of evaluating clinical efficacy.

Some NSAIDs have been associated with undesirable side effects. Although ketoprofen has effective in rats,[31] it has been reported to cause gastrointestinal ulceration.[32,33] There are anecdotal reports of toxicity of carprofen and meloxicam, but such reports are uncommon and the short treatment period required for postoperative pain management is unlikely to result in undesirable side effects. Dosing recommendations for carprofen and meloxicam are usually once daily, but this is based on few data, and twice-daily administration may be required in mice.[34,35] In the rabbit, once-daily administration of meloxicam may be sufficient.[36] In the guinea pig, meloxicam combined with local anesthetic block at the surgical site provided effective pain relief.[7]

Meloxicam is one of the most widely used NSAIDs in small mammals and rabbits in veterinary clinical practice because it is available as both an injectable and palatable oral formulation. The oral formulation is easy to administer to a range of species so can be given to owners to continue analgesic treatment at home.

Acetaminophen (Paracetamol)

Although there are extensive data demonstrating the efficacy of acetaminophen in models of nociception,[37] results when using this agent for postsurgical pain relief have been disappointing (Roughan, personal communication, 2010).[28,38] It is possible that combinations of acetaminophen with NSAIDs or weak opioids may be more effective, but so far few controlled studies have been undertaken for postoperative pain. One attraction of acetaminophen is its availability in a palatable solution,[39] but given its apparent poor efficacy, even at high dose rates, it is usually preferable to administer an NSAID, such as meloxicam.

Opioids

Although there are extensive data on use of a wide range of opioids in rats and mice, the most extensively used agent in these species, and in other small mammals, is buprenorphine.[40] Although this agent is a partial agonist, the degree of analgesia provided is often sufficient to control most postsurgical pain. The duration of action is dose dependent,[41] with higher dose rates providing a longer effect. When administered at the most commonly recommended dose rates (as in **Table 1**), the duration of action may range from 4 hours to 8 hours, depending on the species and the individual.[42–44] This is considerably longer than other opioids, such as morphine, and this prolonged action is largely responsible for the popularity of this agent.

An uncommon side effect of buprenorphine in rats is the onset of pica, which usually manifests as compulsive eating of bedding.[45] This is a nonspecific opioid effect, thought to indicate nausea.[46] If it occurs, then further use of opioids should be avoided in the patient.

Recently a slow-release formulation has become available in the United States, which provides sustained plasma concentrations of buprenorphine for 3 days.[47–49] The slow-release formulation has been shown to have efficacy in several different situations and it may offer an effective means of managing pain, especially when animals are to return home with their owners. One concern is that repeated dosing with buprenorphine for several days has been associated with detrimental effects. This does not seem to occur with slow-release formulations,[43] perhaps because plasma concentrations of the agent are more stable, in contrast to the repeated peaks and troughs associated with intermittent dosing. At present, most data are available for use in rats and mice, but information on pharmacokinetics in other species is being produced.[48] Although many surgical procedures do not result in pain of sufficient intensity and duration to warrant 3 days of opioid administration, if the slow-release formulation can be used without causing undesirable side effects, then it provides a valuable addition to options for pain management in all species.

There is less information on the relative efficacy of other opioids, such as oxymorphone, hydromorphone, butorphanol, and morphine, when used to manage pain in a clinical setting. Laboratory data indicate these opioids are all effective analgesics in rats.[50] They have a shorter duration of action, however, than buprenorphine in small mammals[42] so if used, either frequent repeated dosing is required or analgesia provided using other agents.

Patch formulations of opioids have been used in rabbits, with reports indicating that effective plasma concentrations could be produced, but this was complicated by rapid hair regrowth. Using depilating agents resulted in rapid fentanyl absorption and signs of sedation[51] but with no demonstration of efficacy. Although newer designs of patch can be cut into small pieces to reduce the dose applied, there are no controlled studies of efficacy in small rodent.

Opioids can also be administered epidurally or intrathecally, by percutaneous injection, as in cats and dogs. The technique in rabbits, guinea pigs, and rats is reasonably practicable,[52] although a recent evaluation of intrathecal morphine in rats showed that, unlike in dogs and cats, the duration of action of this opioid was not prolonged when administered by this route.[53] Effective analgesia was, however, produced with a much reduced dose of morphine.

Opioid side effects in small mammals and rabbits rarely cause clinically significant problems. Concern has been expressed that the reduction in gut motility by opioids could be a problem in rabbits, guinea pigs, and chinchillas, because of the sensitivity of these species to postoperative ileus. This does not seem to be a problem in clinical practice. Any effects of opioid administration are likely to be minimal compared with the effects of surgery in producing ileus. In addition, provision of effective pain relief encourages the animals to resume feeding rapidly, and this helps re-establish normal gut function. Finally, if there are concerns about ileus, prokinetics, such as cisapride, can be administered. As an alternative, the H_2 blocker ranitidine has prokinetic properties in rabbits and is often more readily available than cisapride.[54]

Tramadol

Tramadol is a weak opioid with additional analgesic actions by inhibition of serotonin and noradrenaline reuptake, enhancing descending inhibition of nociceptive pathways.[55] The pharmacokinetics of this agent have been studied in rats, mice, and rabbits and efficacy in laboratory models of nociception demonstrated.[56] Studies of its efficacy for postoperative pain management in rats and mice have shown variable efficacy,[57–59] but its good oral bioavailability makes it a potentially useful agent for postoperative analgesia.

Tramadol undergoes rapid metabolism in many species, to a range of metabolites, many of which have analgesic activity. In the rat, the main metabolite is a more potent opioid than tramadol itself.[60] In the rabbit, plasma concentrations of tramadol were low after oral administration[61] and doses recommended for analgesic use (4.4 mg/kg intravenous [IV]) had minimal effects on isoflurane mac.[62] Until clinical efficacy is demonstrated in rabbits, it should be used only when other agents are considered unsuitable.

Because tramadol is available as an oral formulation, it may be suitable for prescribing to provide more prolonged analgesia in animals once they return home, perhaps in combination with an NSAID when more potent analgesia is required.

Local anesthetics

The use of local anesthetics in small mammals has been a neglected option for the provision of postoperative analgesia. This may be due to misinterpretation of some early studies, resulting in statements in textbooks that these agents were highly toxic in rodents. This is clearly not the case. The toxic doses in small rodents, for all the commonly used local anesthetics is similar to that in other species. There are fewer data in rabbits and guinea pigs, but clinical experience and laboratory studies indicate the agents can all be used safely and effectively.

As in other larger species, local anesthetics can be administered as splash blocks, by local infiltration, by blocking specific sensory nerves, and by the epidural or intrathecal route. When using these agents in small mammals, the total safe dosage should be calculated and prepared for use. Although the agents are no more toxic than in other species, the total dose in a 30-g mouse is small (eg, 0.03 mL of 1% lidocaine). When infiltrating a large surgical field (eg, after radical mastectomy in a rat), it is easy to inadvertently overdose. The volume of agent can be increased by dilution, but this reduces the duration of action. Dilutions of lidocaine to 0.25% have been shown to provide effective local block.[63] Lidocaine can also be combined with bupivacaine to provide rapid onset block, followed by prolonged block due to the action of the bupivacaine. Although this approach results in a reduced duration of action of bupivacaine,[64] it is often of considerable clinical benefit by providing effective immediate pain relief. The toxicity of these agents is additive, and in rabbits the recommended maximum dose rates for cats seem appropriate (eg, 1 mg/kg of each agent). In small rodents, higher doses have proved safe and effective in the author's experience (10-mg/kg lidocaine plus 5-mg/kg bupivacaine). Dilution of bupivacaine 1:4 has only a moderate effect on duration of action, so combining the 2 agents in a 50:50 mix and adding an equal volume of water for injection usually provides sufficient volume for infiltration.

Local anesthetic creams, applied topically, are useful for preventing pain during venipuncture[65] and in rabbits provide full-thickness analgesia when applied to the ear.[15]

Preventive Analgesia

Use of preventive analgesia is widely recommended in larger species and the same approach can be used in small mammals. In addition to ensuring pain alleviation is effective in the immediate recovery period, administration of an opioid analgesic as preanesthetic medication potentiates the effects of the anesthetic agents that are administered. This enables effective surgical anesthesia using dose rates of anesthetic that are less depressant to body systems. If volatile agents, such as isoflurane and sevoflurane, are used, then it is easy to adjust the maintenance concentration of anesthetic to allow for this effect. For example, if buprenorphine has been administered 30 minutes to 60 minutes before induction of anesthesia, the maintenance concentration of isoflurane is reduced by approximately 0.5% and sevoflurane by 1%. The induction concentration does not need to be adjusted. Although the time taken to reach a surgical plane of anesthesia is shorter after administration of opioids, this effect is rarely noted in practice. Recovery is not affected but may be smoother because the animal is not experiencing postsurgical pain. It is more difficult to assess the effect when using injectable anesthetic formulations, but in rabbits, there are reports of the use of mixtures of ketamine/medetomidine and either butorphanol or buprenorphine.[66,67] Although these combinations seem safe and effective, the effects are primarily to prolong the duration of anesthesia, and the anesthetic dose sparing effects seen in other species (eg, cats) are not as apparent.

Preoperative administration of NSAIDs does not influence anesthetic depth but can result in more effective postoperative analgesia when administered prior to surgery. One concern is the potentially high incidence of chronic renal disease in small mammals, in particular rabbits and guinea pigs, and especially in older animals. Because preanesthetic assessment of renal function may not be undertaken, it may be safer to delay administration of the NSAID until the end of surgery, during recovery from anesthesia, in animals considered at risk.

Outpatient Analgesia

Although several agents are available that should, when administered at appropriate doses, provide effective analgesia, it can be challenging to extend the period of pain relief if an animal is to be returned home. Returning to the home environment may be beneficial in reducing stress caused by unfamiliar odors, sounds, and noises. It is also important, however, that effective pain relief is provided when necessary. One potentially attractive option is the addition of analgesics to the drinking water, and there are several reports of this approach in a laboratory setting.[68,69] There are several significant problems in using this approach. Small rodents are nocturnal, so little water, and hence little analgesic, is consumed during the day. If the degree of pain relief is ineffective at the end of the day, then animals have a reduced fluid intake. Addition of the analgesic may make the water unpalatable. Rats and guinea pigs are also neophobic, so even if the material is palatable, they may not consume it unless they have been familiarized to the taste previously. Finally, the volume of fluid consumed by small rodents and rabbits varies very considerably between individuals, so the dose of analgesic received also is highly variable. In summary, it is better to provide the owners with a syringe and a small quantity of oral medication, such as meloxicam.

Recommendations

Although it is always important to exercise clinical judgment as to which analgesic regimen is likely to be effective for a particular patient, some general guidance can be suggested. Whichever regimen is selected, it is important to attempt to assess pain to evaluate the efficacy of the analgesics administered.

A typical regimen that is likely to provide effective analgesia after ovariohysterectomy or similar surgery in rabbits or mammary tumor removal in rats is buprenorphine preoperatively, meloxicam or carprofen during recovery from anesthesia, and followed by repeated doses of the NSAID by mouth for the following 1 day to 2 days.[30] If needed, the buprenorphine dosing could be repeated 5 hours to 7 hours after recovery. If prolonged moderate or severe pain is anticipated, then slow-release buprenorphine may be advantageous. Procedures, such as orchiectomy, may not require such prolonged treatment, and use of an opioid together with a single dose of an NSAID might be sufficient. As discussed previously, adding a local anesthetic block seems particularly effective during procedures, such as orchiectomy, where infiltration of the surgical site is easy. To provide both immediate local anesthetic effects, and some postsurgical analgesia, lidocaine should be combined with bupivacaine (or other longer acting local anesthetic).

Managing Other Causes of Pain

Chronic pain may arise from conditions, such as neoplasia, arthritis, and dental disease. Older rodents, in particular rats, commonly develop arthritis, and this may markedly affect their quality of life. Dental disease is also common in rabbits and guinea pigs. Although malocclusion of molar and premolar teeth can be treated surgically, this is a major procedure and may be considered undesirable in specific cases. In these circumstances, control of the associated pain by oral administration of NSAIDs, such as meloxicam, coupled with more conservative dentistry may enable the animal to continue to lead a comfortable life or allow its general clinical condition to be improved before anesthesia and surgery.

As discussed previously, some data exist concerning safety of analgesics in these species, but these assessments are invariably carried out in otherwise healthy, young adult animals. Care, therefore, should be taken when extrapolating these findings to animals that may have preexisting organ damage—for example, chronic renal disease is common in older hamsters, rats, and guinea pigs. This is rarely a significant clinical problem when drugs are used acutely to control postsurgical pain, but special care should be taken if analgesics are administered longer term to manage chronic painful conditions, such as arthritis. Despite these concerns, in the author's experience, oral administration of low doses of NSAIDs for long periods can have positive effects in arthritic rodents. A regimen of 2 weeks to 3 weeks of treatment, followed by a 7-day break, followed by resumption of treatment, reduces the risk of undesirable side effects. Other means of reducing arthritic pain should not be overlooked—feeding of a soft mash, rather than a hard, pelleted diet can improve food intake, especially if arthritis of the mandibular joint is present. Provision of additional soft bedding is also advisable. In addition, consider the design and location of any water bottles, and change these if they require the animal to adopt a posture that could exacerbate joint pain. Anecdotal reports are available regarding the safety of long-term administration of NSAIDs, and it seems that meloxicam can be administered to rabbits for weeks or months at low doses (0.2 mg/kg once a day or twice a day orally) to provide sufficient pain relief to allow animals with dental problems to continue to eat.[70] Adjunctive therapies for arthritis that may be of benefit in other species may also be effective in small mammals. For example, glucosamine/chondroitin has been used in rabbits, with dose rates extrapolated from the cat, and laboratory studies indicate a beneficial effect of glucosamine.[71]

Pain may also arise due to other medical conditions, such as otitis externa, ocular disease, abscesses, and trauma. As in other species, pain should be managed effectively as part of the treatment plan for the condition. Regrettably, analgesic administration may be an afterthought, or completely neglected, when managing conditions where medical treatment is likely to resolve the problem reasonably rapidly. Use of analgesics should always be considered—particularly before undertaking procedures that are likely to exacerbate the degree of pain. For example, administration of an NSAID or even an opioid before attempting to apply topical treatment to otitis externa in a rabbit can be of considerable benefit to the patient.

SUMMARY

Pain in small mammals and rabbits can be managed as effectively as in other species. A range of potentially effective agents is available, and safe dose rates have been established for mice, rats, rabbits, and guinea pigs. Although less information is available of other species, extrapolation between related species often enables safe dosing of less familiar small mammals. New techniques for pain assessment enable evaluation of the efficacy of an analgesic regimen in individual animals, although this remains challenging in a clinical setting.

REFERENCES

1. Gouveia K, Hurst JL. Reducing mouse anxiety during handling: effect of experience with handling tunnels. PLoS One 2013;8(6):e66401. Mintz EM, ed.
2. Hurst JL, West RS. Taming anxiety in laboratory mice. Nat Methods 2010;7(10): 825–6.
3. Roughan JV, Flecknell PA. Behaviour-based assessment of the duration of laparotomy-induced abdominal pain and the analgesic effects of carprofen and buprenorphine in rats. Behav Pharmacol 2004;15(7):461.
4. Wright-Williams S, Flecknell PA, Roughan JV. Comparative effects of vasectomy surgery and buprenorphine treatment on faecal corticosterone concentrations and behaviour assessed by manual and automated analysis methods in C57 and C3H mice. PLoS One 2013;8(9):e75948. Price TJ, ed.
5. Leach MC, Allweiler S, Richardson C, et al. Identifying potential behavioural indicators of pain in rabbits following ovariohysterectomy - preliminary study. Animal Technology and Welfare 2009;8(2):49–52, 70, 74, 78, 82.
6. Leach MC, Allweiler S, Richardson C, et al. Behavioural effects of ovariohysterectomy and oral administration of meloxicam in laboratory housed rabbits. Res Vet Sci 2009;87(2):336–47.
7. Ellen Y, Flecknell P, Leach M. Evaluation of using behavioural changes to assess post-operative pain in the Guinea pig (Cavia porcellus). PLoS One 2016;11(9): e0161941. Pritchett-Corning KR, ed.
8. Liles JH, Flecknell PA. A comparison of the effects of buprenorphine, carprofen and flunixin following laparotomy in rats. J Vet Pharmacol Ther 1994;17(4): 284–90.
9. Arras M, Rettich A, Cinelli P, et al. Assessment of post-laparotomy pain in laboratory mice by telemetric recording of heart rate and heart rate variability. BMC Vet Res 2007;3(1):16.
10. Andrews N, Legg E, Lisak D, et al. Spontaneous burrowing behaviour in the rat is reduced by peripheral nerve injury or inflammation associated pain. Eur J Pain 2012;16(4):485–95.
11. Jirkof P. Burrowing and nest building behavior as indicators of well-being in mice. J Neurosci Methods 2014;234:139–46.
12. Darwin C. The expression of emotion in man and animals. London: Penguin; 2009.
13. Langford DJ, Bailey AL, Chanda ML, et al. Coding of facial expressions of pain in the laboratory mouse. Nat Methods 2010;7(6):447–9.
14. Sotocinal SG, Sorge RE, Zaloum A, et al. The rat grimace scale: a partially automated method for quantifying pain in the laboratory rat via facial expressions. Mol Pain 2011;7(1):55.
15. Keating SCJ, Thomas AA, Flecknell PA, et al. Evaluation of EMLA cream for preventing pain during tattooing of rabbits: changes in physiological, behavioural and facial expression responses. PLoS One 2012;7(9):e44437.
16. Costa ED, Minero M, Lebelt D, et al. Development of the horse grimace scale (HGS) as a pain assessment tool in horses undergoing routine castration. PLoS One 2014;9(3):e92281. Hillman E, ed.

17. McLennan KM, Rebelo CJB, Corke MJ, et al. Development of a facial expression scale using footrot and mastitis as models of pain in sheep. Appl Anim Behav Sci 2016;176:19–26.
18. Guesgen MJ, Beausoleil NJ, Leach M, et al. Coding and quantification of a facial expression for pain in lambs. Behav Processes 2016;132:49–56.
19. Di Giminiani P, Brierley VLMH, Scollo A, et al. The assessment of facial expressions in piglets undergoing tail docking and castration: toward the development of the piglet grimace scale. Front Vet Sci 2016;3:261.
20. Descovich KA, Wathan J, Leach MC, et al. Facial expression: an under-utilised tool for the assessment of welfare in mammals. ALTEX 2017;34(3):409–29.
21. Defensor EB, Corley MJ, Blanchard RJ, et al. Facial expressions of mice in aggressive and fearful contexts. Physiol Behav 2012;107(5):680–5.
22. Oliver V, De Rantere D, Ritchie R, et al. Psychometric assessment of the rat grimace scale and development of an analgesic intervention score. PLoS One 2014;9(5):e97882. McCormick C, ed.
23. Leung V, Zhang E, Pang DS. Real-time application of the rat grimace Scale as a welfare refinement in laboratory rats. Sci Rep 2016;6(1):31667.
24. Flecknell P. Laboratory animal anaesthesia. London: Academic Press; 2015.
25. Hawkins MG. The use of analgesics in birds, reptiles, and small exotic mammals. Journal of exotic pet medicine 2006;15(3):177–92.
26. Wright-Willams S, Courade J, Richardson C, et al. Effects of vasectomy surgery and meloxicam treatment on faecal corticosterone levels and behaviour in two strains of laboratory mouse. Pain 2007;130(1–2):108–18.
27. Miller AL, Roughan JV. A comparison of abdominal and scrotal approach methods of vasectomy and the influence of analgesic treatment in laboratory mice. Lab Anim 2012;46(4):304–10.
28. Matsumiya LC, Sorge RE, Sotocinal SG, et al. Using the mouse grimace scale to reevaluate the efficacy of postoperative analgesics in laboratory mice. J Am Assoc Lab Anim Sci 2012;51(1):42–9.
29. Cooper CS, Metcalf-Pate KA, Barat CE, et al. Comparison of side effects between buprenorphine and meloxicam used postoperatively in Dutch belted rabbits (Oryctolagus cuniculus). J Am Assoc Lab Anim Sci 2009;48(3):279–85.
30. Goldschlager GB, Gillespie VL, Palme R, et al. Effects of multimodal analgesia with lowdose buprenorphine and meloxicam on fecal glucocorticoid metabolites after surgery in New Zealand white rabbits (Oryctolagus cuniculus). J Am Assoc Lab Anim Sci 2013;52(5):571–6.
31. Roughan JV, Flecknell PA. Behavioural effects of laparotomy and analgesic effects of ketoprofen and carprofen in rats. Pain 2001;90(1):65–74.
32. Lamon TK, Browder EJ, Sohrabji F, et al. Adverse effects of incorporating ketoprofen into established rodent studies. J Am Assoc Lab Anim Sci 2008;47(4):20–4.
33. Shientag LJ, Wheeler SM, Garlick DS, et al. A therapeutic dose of ketoprofen causes acute gastrointestinal bleeding, erosions, and ulcers in rats. J Am Assoc Lab Anim Sci 2012;51(6):832–41.
34. Engelhardt G, Homma D, Schlegel K, et al. General pharmacology of meloxicam-part I: effects on CNS, gastric emptying, intestinal transport, water, electrolyte and creatinine excretion. Gen Pharmacol 1996;27(4):673–7. Available at: http://www.sciencedirect.com/science/article/pii/0306362395020349.
35. Busch U, Schmid J, Heinzel G, et al. Pharmacokinetics of meloxicam in animals and the relevance to humans. Drug Metab Dispos 1998;26(6):576–84. Available at: http://dmd.aspetjournals.org/content/26/6/576.short.

36. Turner PV, Chen HC, Taylor WM. Pharmacokinetics of meloxicam in rabbits after single and repeat oral dosing. Comp Med 2006;56(1):63–7. Available at: http://eutils.ncbi.nlm.nih.gov/entrez/eutils/elink.fcgi?dbfrom=pubmed&id=16521861&retmode=ref&cmd=prlinks.

37. Miranda HF, Puig MM, Prieto JC, et al. Synergism between paracetamol and nonsteroidal anti-inflammatory drugs in experimental acute pain. Pain 2006; 121(1–2):22–8.

38. Dickinson AL, Leach MC, Flecknell PA. The analgesic effects of oral paracetamol in two strains of mice undergoing vasectomy. Lab Anim 2009;43(4): 357–61.

39. Fleischmann T, Arras M, Sauer M, et al. Voluntary intake of paracetamol-enriched drinking water and its influence on the success of embryo transfer in mice. Res Vet Sci 2017;111:85–92.

40. Stokes EL, Flecknell PA, Richardson CA. Reported analgesic and anaesthetic administration to rodents undergoing experimental surgical procedures. Lab Anim 2009;43(2):149–54.

41. Roughan JV, Flecknell PA. Buprenorphine: a reappraisal of its antinociceptive effects and therapeutic use in alleviating post-operative pain in animals. Lab Anim 2002;36(3):322–43.

42. Gades NM, Danneman PJ, Wixson SK, et al. The magnitude and duration of the analgesic effect of morphine, butorphanol, and buprenorphine in rats and mice. Contemp Top Lab Anim Sci 2000;39(2):8–13.

43. Jirkof P, Tourvieille A, Cinelli P, et al. Buprenorphine for pain relief in mice: repeated injections vs sustained-release depot formulation. Lab Anim 2015; 49(3):177–87.

44. Sauer M, Fleischmann T, Lipiski M, et al. Buprenorphine via drinking water and combined oral-injection protocols for pain relief in mice. Appl Anim Behav Sci 2016;185:103–12.

45. Clark JA, Myers PH, Goelz MF, et al. Pica behavior associated with buprenorphine administration in the rat. Lab Anim Sci 1997;47(3):300–3.

46. Batra VR, Schrott LM. Acute oxycodone induces the pro-emetic pica response in rats. J Pharmacol Exp Ther 2011;339(3):738–45.

47. Kendall LV, Wegenast DJ, Smith BJ, et al. Efficacy of sustained-release buprenorphine in an experimental laparotomy model in female mice. J Am Assoc Lab Anim Sci 2016;55(1):66–73.

48. DiVincenti L, Meirelles LAD, Westcott RA. Safety and clinical effectiveness of a compounded sustained-release formulation of buprenorphine for postoperative analgesia in New Zealand white rabbits. J Am Vet Med Assoc 2016;248(7): 795–801.

49. Foley PL. Evaluation of a sustained-release formulation of buprenorphine for analgesia in rats. J Am Assoc Lab Anim Sci 2011;50(2):198–204.

50. Peckham EM, Traynor JR. Comparison of the antinociceptive response to morphine and morphine-like compounds in male and female sprague-dawley rats. J Pharmacol Exp Ther 2006;316(3):1195–201.

51. Foley PL, Henderson AL, Bissonette EA, et al. Evaluation of fentanyl transdermal patches in rabbits: blood concentrations and physiologic response. Comp Med 2001;51(3):239–44.

52. Turner PV, Brabb T, Pekow C, et al. Administration of substances to laboratory animals: routes of administration and factors to consider. J Am Assoc Lab Anim Sci 2011;50(5):600–13.

53. Thomas A, Miller A, Roughan J, et al. Efficacy of intrathecal morphine in a model of surgical pain in rats. PLoS One 2016;11(10):e0163909–21. Bader M, ed.

54. Wenger S. Anesthesia and analgesia in rabbits and rodents. Journal of exotic pet medicine 2012;21(1):7–16.

55. Raffa RB, Friderichs E, Reimann W, et al. Opioid and nonopioid components independently contribute to the mechanism of action of tramadol, an "atypical" opioid analgesic. J Pharmacol Exp Ther 1992;260(1):275–85.

56. Oyama T, Homan T, Kyotani J, et al. Effect of tramadol on pain-related behaviors and bladder overactivity in rodent cystitis models. Eur J Pharmacol 2012; 676(1–3):75–80.

57. Zegre Cannon C, Kissling GE, Goulding DR, et al. Analgesic effects of tramadol, carprofen or multimodal analgesia in rats undergoing ventral laparotomy. Lab Anim (NY) 2011;40(3):85–93.

58. Wolfe AM, Kennedy LH, Na JJ, et al. Efficacy of tramadol as a sole analgesic for postoperative pain in male and female mice. J Am Assoc Lab Anim Sci 2015; 54(4):411–9.

59. Taylor BF, Ramirez HE, Battles AH, et al. Analgesic activity of tramadol and buprenorphine after voluntary ingestion by rats (Rattus norvegicus). J Am Assoc Lab Anim Sci 2016;55(1):74–82.

60. Valle M, Garrido MJ, Pavón JM, et al. Pharmacokinetic-pharmacodynamic modeling of the antinociceptive effects of main active metabolites of tramadol, (+)-O-desmethyltramadol and (-)-O-desmethyltramadol, in rats. J Pharmacol Exp Ther 2000;293(2):646–53.

61. Souza MJ, Cox SK. Pharmacokinetics of orally administered tramadol in domestic rabbits (Oryctolagus cuniculus). Am J Vet Res 2008;69(8):979–82.

62. Egger CM, Souza MJ, Greenacre CB, et al. Effect of intravenous administration of tramadol hydrochloride on the minimum alveolar concentration of isoflurane in rabbits. Am J Vet Res 2009;70(8):945–9.

63. Grant GJ, Piskoun B, Lin A, et al. An in vivo method for the quantitative evaluation of local anesthetics. J Pharmacol Toxicol Methods 2000;43(1):69–72.

64. Cuvillon P, Nouvellon E, Ripart J, et al. A comparison of the pharmacodynamics and pharmacokinetics of bupivacaine, ropivacaine (with epinephrine) and their equal volume mixtures with lidocaine used for femoral and sciatic nerve blocks: a double-blind randomized study. Anesth Analg 2009;108(2): 641–9.

65. Flecknell PA, Liles JH, Williamson HA. The use of lignocaine-prilocaine local anaesthetic cream for pain-free venepuncture in laboratory animals. Lab Anim 1990;24(2):142–6.

66. Hedenqvist P, Orr HE, Roughan JV, et al. Anaesthesia with ketamine/medetomidine in the rabbit: influence of route of administration and the effect of combination with butorphanol. Vet Anaesth Analg 2002;29(1):14–9.

67. Murphy KL, Baxter MG, Flecknell PA. Anaesthesia with a combination of ketamine and medetomidine in the rabbit: effect of premedication with buprenorphine. Vet Anaesth Analg 2010;37(3):222–9.

68. Mickley GA, Hoxha Z, Biada JM, et al. Acetaminophen self-administered in the drinking water increases the pain threshold of rats (Rattus norvegicus). J Am Assoc Lab Anim Sci 2006;45(5):48–54. Available at: http://eutils.ncbi.nlm.nih.gov/entrez/eutils/elink.fcgi?dbfrom=pubmed&id=16995647&retmode=ref&cmd=prlinks.

69. Speth RC, Smith MS, Brogan RS. Regarding the inadvisability of administering postoperative analgesics in the drinking water of rats (Rattus norvegicus). Contemp Top Lab Anim Sci 2001;40(6):15–7.

70. Harcourt-Brown F. Textbook of rabbit medicine. Oxford (UK): Butterworth-Heine-mann Medical; 2002.
71. Tiraloche G, Girard C, Chouinard L, et al. Effect of oral glucosamine on cartilage degradation in a rabbit model of osteoarthritis. Arthritis Rheum 2005;52(4): 1118–28.

Vaccination of Ferrets for Rabies and Distemper

Laura L. Wade, DVM, DABVP (Avian)

KEYWORDS

- Ferret • Rabies • Distemper • Virus • Vaccine

KEY POINTS

- Companion ferrets need to be vaccinated against 2 viral diseases that cause neurologic illness: canine distemper and rabies.
- Both viruses are fatal in ferrets, and rabies virus is fatal in humans.
- All ferrets that are used for hunting, take walks in public places, or are taken to shows should be vaccinated for distemper. Distemper virus does not live long outside the host and is transmitted by close contact with an infected animal.

Companion ferrets need to be vaccinated against 2 viral diseases that cause neurologic illness: canine distemper and rabies. Although not common in ferrets, both viruses are fatal in ferrets, and rabies virus is fatal in humans.

An excellent review of these and other viral diseases in ferrets was published in a previous edition of *Veterinary Clinics of North America: Exotic Animal Practice* and the latest edition of *Biology and Diseases of the Ferret*.[1,2] Readers can review diseases of the central nervous system, including rabies and distemper, in recent texts.[3–6] In this article, we provide a basic review of the 2 diseases and update current vaccine concerns from a practitioner's perspective. Additional information regarding vaccine wellness can be found in current texbooks.[7–9]

DISTEMPER

Canine distemper virus (CDV) is an RNA virus in the genus *Morbillivirus* in the Paramyxoviridae family. It displays one of the highest incidences of central nervous system involvement within the *Morbillivirus* genus. CDV is closely related to measles virus (MV) that infects humans, although ferrets cannot be infected with MV. Spread by aerosolization, ferrets infected with CDV typically develop a clinical course comparable to measles, which includes upper respiratory signs and fever, followed by a fatal neurotropic phase. Affected ferrets develop a severe leukopenia (lymphopenia), which

The author has nothing to disclose.
Specialized Care for Avian & Exotic Pets, 10882 Main Street, Clarence, NY 14031, USA
E-mail address: buffalobirdnerd@gmail.com

vetexotic.theclinics.com

is the hallmark of *Morbillivirus* infections. Some ferrets will develop loss of appetite and diarrhea.

Similar to dogs, ferrets develop a more serious course of cutaneous lesions, such as an erythematous, pruritic papular rash that begins on the chin and spreads to the inguinal area. Inconsistently, they also may develop hyperkeratosis of the planum nasale and footpad. Affected ferrets also may develop oculonasal discharge associated with rhinitis and lower airway disease, such as pneumonia. Several references show excellent pictures of these external lesions.[10,11] The neurotropic phase includes hyperexcitability, muscle tremors, hypersalivation, paresis, coma, and death. Ferrets that die within 2 weeks of sepsis and multiorgan failure do not typically develop neurologic signs. In contrast, neurotropic strains cause disease lasting 3 to 5 weeks with the classic chewing gum seizures and head pressing. Disease duration is the main neurovirulence determinant, and when infected with a neurovirulent strain, most ferrets will develop neurologic signs that increase with disease progression.[12] The classic presentation of CDV in ferrets has its exceptions, however: there is a report of a previously vaccinated ferret that presented for dermatologic lesions and prolonged course (3 weeks) with the absence of respiratory and neurologic signs.[13] The investigators note that CDV should remain a clinical suspicion for ferrets with skin lesions that do not respond to appropriate therapy, even in animals that were previously vaccinated.

Distemper is nearly 100% fatal in ferrets that become infected and there is no effective treatment.[14] Sources of infection are usually pet dogs in the house, foxes (ferrets that go outside), and other ferrets. All ferrets that are used for hunting, take walks in public places, or are taken to shows should be vaccinated for distemper. Distemper virus does not live long outside the host and is transmitted by close contact with an infected animal; however, vaccination before exposure is the only way to protect ferrets from infection.

Ferrets are excellent models for evaluating the ability of CDV vaccines to protect against symptomatic infection.[14] In the past decade, available approved and "off-label" vaccines for ferrets have been lost and gained. Currently, the only vaccine licensed for ferrets is Merial's Purevax (**Table 1**). Since 2001, this nonadjuvanted, lyophilized vaccine of a recombinant canary pox vector that expresses glycoproteins

Table 1
Vaccines available for use in ferrets in the United States

Virus	Vaccine	Manufacturer	Virus Viability	Licensed for Ferrets	Label Schedule	Booster
Rabies	IMRAB 3 IMRAB 3 TF[a]	Merial, Inc (Duluth, GA)	Killed	YES	>12 wk	Annual
	Defensor 1 Defensor 3	Zoetis Inc (Parsippany, NJ)	Killed	YES	>3 mo	Annual
	Nobivac 1 Nobivac 3	Zoetis Inc (Parsippany, NJ)	Killed	YES (except CA)	>3 mo	Annual
Distemper	PUREVAX[a]	Merial, Inc (Duluth, GA)	Live Canarypox Vector Recombinant	YES	>8 wk	3 and 6 wk, then annual
	Nobivac Puppy-DPv[a]	Intervet/Merck Animal Health (Madison, NJ)	Modified live vaccine	NO	See text	See text

[a] Thimersol-free.

of CDV has become the preferred distemper vaccine. Previously, Fervac D (United Vaccines, Madison, WI), a modified live virus vaccine of chick cell origin licensed for ferrets in North America, was used but is no longer available. Studies show use of recombinant poxvirus vaccines (vs attenuated CDV vaccines) is a possible method of overcoming interference of maternally acquired antibody.[15]

Because the Purevax vaccine has been on intermittent backorder over the past several years, many exotic animal veterinarians in the United States have been using the modified live Nobivac DPv canine distemper-parvovirus (Intervet/Merck, Madison, NJ) "off-label" to protect ferrets (see **Table 1**). In the United States, according to the American Veterinary Medical Association, veterinarians can use a vaccine that is not approved for ferrets.[16] According the manufacturer, a similar vaccine has been used in the United Kingdom "off-label" in ferrets and mink with no reported problems. Feedback and field experience have shown the vaccine is tolerated well.[7] The author has used the Nobivac DPv in her clinic and also found it to be tolerated well with no serious side effects over a period of several years. Purevax is the recommended vaccine from the American Ferret Association (AFA).[17] In our clinic, we prefer to use the Merial Purevax vaccine as approved for ferrets. If/when Purevax is on backorder, Nobivac DPv is used.

Probably the most challenging aspect of vaccinating has occurred in the past few years regarding boosters. When to give, and how many to give? Since 2013, The AFA recommends the vaccine schedule should begin at 8 weeks of age, followed by booster vaccinations at 11 and 14 weeks, and an annual booster.[17] More specifically, for healthy kits 14 weeks of age or younger from mothers whose vaccination history is unknown, incomplete, or outdated, or for kits that have had unknown, incomplete, or no vaccination history, give a series of 3 vaccinations, 3 weeks apart, with annual boosters. For healthy ferrets older than 14 weeks that have unknown, incomplete, outdated, or no vaccination history: give a series of 2 vaccinations, 3 weeks apart with annual boosters thereafter.[18]

Initial vaccine in most ferrets in the United States (Marshall Farms, North Rose, NY) is given at the facility using a mink vaccine at 5 weeks of age. Full immune response requires boosters to complete protection, a system similar to what is done with puppies. However, maternal antibody interferes before 10 weeks and may do so up until 16 weeks of age.[19,20] The most important thing to remember is that ferrets must have at least 2 vaccines for immunity to develop. In the simplest form, this means a young ferret with low risk should be vaccinated at 10 to 12 and 14 to 16 weeks if a previous vaccine has been given. Young ferrets with increased risks (pet stores, face of an outbreak) should be started at 6 to 8 weeks of age, continued every 3 weeks until 16 weeks. Any ferret with unknown history (whether or not tattoo is present), should receive 2 distemper vaccines 3 to 4 weeks apart (C. Johnson-Delaney, 2016, oral communication).[19] In light of this, our current general recommendation for clients with young ferrets is a booster as soon as the ferret is purchased, and then every 3 weeks until they are 16 weeks of age. Young ferrets should be keep in isolation for 2 weeks after the last vaccination (C. Johnson-Delaney, 2016, oral communication).

Although Merial (Duluth, GA) recommends boosters yearly, there is some question to the possibility that immunity may last much longer. Recent research has shown that if ferrets receive their first vaccine before 9 weeks of age and a booster at 14 to 16 weeks, 90% have protection for at least 3 years.[21] After the initial series, antibody titers can be done to see if subsequent vaccines need to be given. The AFA suggests using a serum neutralization titer (minimum of 100 µL serum) through Cornell University College of Veterinary Medicine (Ithaca, NY).[20] Titers greater than 1:50 are considered protective and no booster is needed, but sometimes ferrets do not make a good antibody response to a vaccine. This makes them susceptible to infection. Ferrets with titers less than 1:50 should receive a booster (exceptions, see vaccine reactions later in this article).[21]

There have been several recent outbreaks of distemper in vaccinated ferrets in rescues and shelters.[7,21] Ferrets with up-to-date vaccinations have died and ferrets with out-of-date vaccinations did not experience signs; however, most ferrets that were vaccinated did not show signs of disease or survived with minor effects. Contrary to Wagner and Bhardwaj,[21] a study by Pavlacik and colleagues[22] showed poor antibody induction with several modified live vaccines (MLVs) commonly used for puppies at 6, 10, and 14 weeks. The major difference between these articles is that all vaccines used in Wagner and Bhardwaj[21] were MLVs, whereas Pavlacik and colleagues[22] had a mixture of killed and MLVs. Pavlacik and colleagues[22] admit that inactivated CDV has unreliable efficacy.

In light of all these possibilities, a risk assessment should be done at the initial and annual physical examinations. Ferrets that are taken outside, to pet stores, boarding facilities, or if their titers are low may need to be boosted yearly. Ferrets that live indoors, do not travel, or have adequate titers, may be boosted every 3 years. All clients should receive education on distemper virus and vaccination. A good, albeit slightly outdated (available vaccines) veterinarian-written client handout can be obtained online.[23]

RABIES

Rhabdovirus is a neurotropic RNA virus in the genus *Lyssavirus*. In mammals, rabies causes an acute, progressive encephalitis. Infection occurs primarily from contact with infected saliva from a bite wound from a rabid animal. In ferrets, rabies is an acute and almost invariably fatal disease that is also zoonotic. Clinical signs are ascending paralysis, ataxia, tremors, paresthesia, hyperactivity, anorexia, cachexia, bladder atony, tremors, fever, and hypothermia. Shedding of virus in the saliva is variable and dependent on the variant of virus exposed.

In the United States, canine rabies virus has been eliminated, but skunk, bat, fox, and raccoon variants exist in wild mammal populations. Exposure to bats and foxes could be a source of infection, as well as unvaccinated dogs and cats. Incubation periods have been shown to be dependent on viral dose. Exposure to rabies virus does not always lead to infection, but once clinical signs are evident, the disease is almost always fatal.[24,25] A recent report of a ferret experimentally infected with skunk-origin rabies developed hind limb paralysis but survived with paraplegia.[26]

Rabies is rare in vaccinated animals.[27] If a nonvaccinated ferret bites a person, the health department may require it to be quarantined for observation or be euthanized and tested for rabies. According to the Centers for Disease Control and Prevention, no person in the United States has ever contracted rabies from a dog cat or ferret held in quarantine for 10 days.[28] To travel to Canada or other foreign countries, ferrets must have proof of rabies vaccination or an exemption certificate (see vaccine reactions later in this article). Before interstate movement occurs, ferrets should be vaccinated. A useful form from the National Association of State Public Health Veterinarians is available online.[29]

Until recently, Merial IMRAB 3 and IMRAB 3 TF were the only rabies vaccines approved for ferrets. In 1984, IMRAB 3 was licensed for ferrets and comes in a multidose vial. In 2002, the thimerosal-free, individual-dose vaccine was approved for ferrets (see **Table 1**). In February 2017, Zoetis (Parsippany, NJ) obtained license approval in all states except California for a new rabies vaccine for ferrets, labeled as Defensor 1 and Defensor 3 (see **Table 1**). According to the manufacturer, the 2 products are identical and the label claim extension applies only to dogs and cats for Defensor 3. Efficacy was confirmed in a 1-year duration of immunity study in which none of the vaccinated animals were infected with rabies when challenged 12 months after a single dose of Defensor. During a field safety study conducted in 200 ferrets, no significant postvaccination reactions were observed.[30] In March 2017, Nobivac 1 and Nobivac 3 were approved for ferrets by Merck/Intervet. These vaccines are identical to the Defensor 1 and 3 vaccines and are manufactured by Zoetis (see **Table 1**).

In all of the rabies vaccines, the initial vaccine should be given at 12 weeks or older with boosters annually. Ferrets are considered immunized if the primary vaccination was administered at least 28 days previously.[27] Regardless of the age of the animal at initial vaccination, a booster vaccination should be administered 1 year later.[27] Imrab vaccine was shown to protect up to 90% of ferrets exposed to rabies for up to 1 year.[31]

Rabies titers are not commercially validated or accepted. In ferrets that develop anaphylaxis, determining if they are immune competent while carrying a protective titer still might be useful. Serologic titers also can be used to identify potentially susceptible animals (negative titer). Risk assessment should be made and if deemed low risk of exposure, an exemption certificate may be written by the veterinarian. This would be important to keep on hand and should accompany the traveling ferret.

If a ferret has not been vaccinated and is exposed to a known rabid animal, the ferret should be humanely euthanized immediately or quarantined for 6 months. Those that are euthanized will need to have their brains tested by an appropriate laboratory for rabies. For those that are quarantined, the 6-month quarantine is required, as there is evidence that the use of vaccine alone will not reliably prevent disease when vaccinated after exposure. Ferrets that are current on vaccination should receive veterinary medical care immediately for assessment, wound cleansing, and booster vaccination. The ferret should be kept under its owner's care for 45 days of observation. Ferrets that are overdue for a rabies vaccine should be evaluated on a case-by-case basis to determine the need for euthanasia or immediate booster vaccination followed by quarantine.[28]

VACCINE REACTIONS

Type 1 hypersensitivity reactions manifest in redness of the skin, restlessness, respiratory distress, vomiting, diarrhea, bleeding, collapse, and sometimes, death. Typically, allergic reactions occur within the first 30 minutes, but may occur up to 8 hours after vaccination. Vaccine reactions have been reported as more common after distemper vaccination but also occur with rabies vaccination (see details that follow). Multiple vaccinations with modified live virus vaccines are associated with a high incidence of vaccine-induced adverse reactions, especially anaphylaxis.[32,33] Merial's nonadjuvanted, incomplete distemper protein has 0.3% reaction according to the company, which is much lower than the previously available Fervac D (5.9%).[32]

There are 2 studies in the past 15 years that provide conflicting results. Greenacre[32] showed a significant overall vaccine reaction (9%). Of these cases, distemper vaccination and the administration of 2 vaccines significantly increased the risk of reaction (71% reaction to both vaccines vs 21% only distemper and 7% only rabies). Ferrets that had an anaphylactic reaction were significantly older at the time of vaccination than ferrets that did not react.[32] Another retrospective study with a larger number of ferrets showed a much smaller percentage of reactions (0.8%). The difference in incidences among vaccines (1% reaction to distemper, 0.85% reaction to rabies and distemper, and 0.51% reaction to rabies) was not considered significant. In this study, although age was not a significant risk factor, the risk of reaction increased by 80% with each successive distemper vaccination.[33] No specific vaccine component has been shown to be responsible for the hypersensitivity. Hypersensitization is thought to be long-lived, but repeatability cannot be presumed. Several ferrets that had reactions were revaccinated without adverse event.[33]

There are 8 reports of vaccine-associated fibrosarcoma in ferrets, and it was not determined which vaccine caused the reaction in all cases.[34,35] One study[35] described 5 of 7 ferrets with vaccination site fibrosarcomas (VSFs) that had received a rabies vaccine within the previous 12 months. Three of these ferrets also received vaccinations against canine distemper within a year of developing VSF. The investigators indicate that rabies vaccine is considered more likely to contribute to VSFs than distemper vaccine.[35] The author of the present article had a case of severe granulomatous reaction that developed 1 year after initial distemper vaccine series (2 doses of Merial Purevax were given 1 month apart in the location of the granuloma), which responded with surgical removal. This ferret received a rabies vaccine in another location during the same time period the previous year. The report with the 7 ferrets with VSFs did not detail which vaccine was given where,[35] and in the report with the single ferret, both vaccines were given at the VSF site.[34] Veterinarians should be consistent in their vaccine administration sites. The author routinely gives distemper in the right scapular region and rabies in the right hip region. This way, if any local abnormalities develop, the causative vaccine could be determined.

RISK ASSESSMENT AND VACCINATION POLICY

Annual examination and client lifestyle evaluation is important for risk assessment. We believe that the first vaccines a ferret gets are probably the most important. Just like with vaccinating dogs and cats for serious diseases, the immunity obtained can be life-saving; however, ferrets may have adverse reactions to vaccines more often than dogs and cats. Risks of vaccines, including allergic reaction (more common) and injection site fibrosarcoma (rare), should be discussed. Lethargy (sleeping) and tenderness to the touch (vaccine site) are considered normal postvaccine reactions and should resolve within 12 to 24 hours.

At our hospital, we recommend a minimum of 25 minutes of observation after vaccination.[32] We want to know if a problem is happening while the ferret is still in the clinic. We give an oral dose of diphenhydramine before giving vaccines (0.5 mL of Children's Benadryl [2.5 mg/mL; Johnson & Johnson, New Brunswick, NJ] for ferrets up to 1 kg, 0.6–0.75 mL for ferrets heavier than 1 kg) as a precaution.[21] If a reaction occurs, a different medication for allergic reactions (intravenous dexamethasone, epinephrine with possible fluid administration) will be administered immediately and most ferrets recover. An important reminder is that diphenhydramine can cause sleepiness or hyperexcitability and may mask a reaction.

We do not advise vaccinating ferrets at "free rabies clinics" unless the veterinarian is prepared to treat an allergic reaction (must have injectable diphenhydramine on hand and willing to be available for 30 minutes after vaccination).

Only 1 vaccine should be given at a time to reduce antigen load on the immune system and to determine which vaccine might play a role in a reaction, if any develop. Therefore, rabies and distemper vaccines are administered separately, with the other vaccine administered 2 to 4 weeks later. Distemper boosters are administered 3 to 4 weeks after the first initial distemper vaccine.

Ferrets that board at our hospital must have proof of vaccination (distemper vaccine or appropriate titer within 1 year and rabies vaccine within 1 year unless exempt due to a vaccine reaction). Ferrets that are hospitalized should have similar proof of vaccination. Sick ferrets with an unknown vaccine history may be placed into isolation for the safety of other ferrets in the hospital even though we do not treat dogs or rabies vector wildlife at our hospital.

Our wellness program for new kits and adult ferrets is shown as follows. The adult ferret schedule assumes incomplete or unknown previous health history. A useful chart to help clients keep track of their ferret's vaccine schedule is shown in **Table 2**.

Ideal Kit Wellness and Vaccine Schedule

Examination, distemper vaccine, fecal float, and ear mite check performed at 9 to 12 weeks.
Three to 4 weeks later: examination/distemper vaccine at 12 to 16 weeks.
One week later (or as required depending on state or county requirements), rabies vaccine.
Subsequent boosters: rabies annual, distemper (or vaccine titer) every 1 to 3 years (or as indicated through risk assessment).

Ideal Adult Ferret Wellness Vaccine Schedule

Examination, fecal float, ear mite check, distemper vaccine given or titer drawn.
Examination, distemper booster 3 to 4 weeks later if unknown vaccine history or low titer.
Rabies vaccine given 1 to 2 weeks later.
Subsequent boosters: rabies annual, distemper (or vaccine titer) every 1 to 3 years (or as indicated through risk assessment).

Table 2
Client education chart: "My Ferret's Vaccine Schedule (First 5 years)"

	When Due	Date Given	Postvaccine Observations
1st year vaccines			
Distemper 1			
Distemper 2			
Distemper 3			
Rabies			
2nd year vaccines			
Distemper			
Rabies			
3rd year vaccines			
Distemper			
Rabies			
4th year vaccines			
Distemper			
Rabies			
5th year vaccines			
Distemper			
Rabies			

Protocol and Strategies for Ferrets that Develop a Vaccine Reaction

If a ferret develops signs of an allergic reaction (gastrointestinal or respiratory distress or extreme weakness/collapse), the vaccine that caused the reaction should not be administered in the future and a warning placed in the medical record. This is especially important for low-risk patients. If the reaction is to distemper vaccine, a distemper antibody titer may be performed to assess level of protection. Ferrets with low titers should be considered at risk and should be allowed only around dogs and ferrets that are vaccinated adequately for distemper. If the ferret is high risk, administration of one-tenth to one-half the dose can be administered to reduce the concentration product.[36,37] Another option might be to use an alternate vaccine (give Nobivac DPv to ferret that reacts to Purevax) with close supervision and administration of an antihistamine. A ferret that reacts to one vaccine may or may not react to another. However, consider an abundance of caution, and diphenhydramine should be administered via intramuscular injection (1 mg/kg) before administering another vaccine and the ferret should be monitored for a minimum of 30 minutes or longer. Ferrets that have a reaction to a rabies vaccine should have an exemption certificate written by the veterinarian in case of travel.

THE FERRET AND VACCINE DEVELOPMENT OF THE FUTURE

Because ferrets have such a high sensitivity to CDV, they are an attractive animal model for the study of *Morbillivirus* disease, vaccines, and treatments.[14,38] Ferrets are excellent models for the development of vaccines for vulnerable populations of carnivores and humans. Most notably, active research focuses on the development of gene therapy vectors and recombinant vaccine platforms. A recent study showed a bivalent rabies virus–based vaccine against CDV induces protective immune responses against both pathogens. The researchers generated recombinant inactivated rabies viruses that carry one of the CDV glycoproteins on their surface.[39]

Another strategy that has not been studied in ferrets, but has worked well in other species might include using one vaccine for the priming and another for the booster. By presenting the antigen in a different format, the immune system can thus be stimulated. An example of this would be to use Purevax for initial vaccine, with Nobivac for the booster. In this way, an early, safe immunization in the face of maternal antibodies can be obtained, and a substantial boost follows with the subsequent modified live version (E.J. Dubovi, 2017, oral communication).

ACKNOWLEDGMENTS

I would like to thank Cathy A. Johnson-Delaney, DVM (Washington Ferret Rescue & Shelter, Kirkland, WA) and Edward J. Dubovi, PhD (Virology Laboratory, Animal Health Diagnostic Center, College of Veterinary Medicine, Cornell University, Ithaca, NY) for substantial contributions to this article's development and revision.

REFERENCES

1. Langlois I. Viral diseases of ferrets. Vet Clin North Am Exot Anim Pract 2005;8(1): 139–60.
2. Kiupel M, Perpinan D. Viral diseases of ferrets. Biology and diseases of the ferret. 3rd edition. Ames (IA): John Wiley & Sons; 2014. p. 439–517.
3. Tully TN. Central nervous system. In: Mitchell MA, Tully TN, editors. Current therapy in exotic pet practice. St Louis (MO): Elsevier; 2016. p. 392–434.

4. Fox JG. Other systemic diseases. Biology and diseases of the ferret. 3rd edition. Ames (IA): John Wiley & Sons; 2014. p. 421–38.
5. Orosz SW, Johnson-Delaney CA. Disorders of the nervous system. In: Johnson-Delaney CA, editor. Ferret medicine surgery. Boca Raton (FL): CRC Press; 2016. p. 273–88.
6. Antinoff NM, Giovanella CJ. Musculoskeletal and neurologic diseases. In: Quesenberry KE, Carpenter JW, editors. Ferrets, rabbits and rodents clinical medicine and surgery. 3rd edition. St Louis (MO): Elsevier; 2012. p. 132–40.
7. Chitty JR, Johnson-Delaney CA. Ferret preventive care. In: Johnson-Delaney CA, editor. Ferret medicine and surgery. Boca Raton (FL). CRC Press; 2016. p. 85–93.
8. Marini RP. Physical examination, preventive medicine and diagnosis in the ferret. In: Fox JG, Marini RP, editors. Biology and diseases of the ferret. 3rd edition. Ames (IA): John Wiley & Sons; 2014. p. 235–58.
9. Quesenberry KE, Orcutt C. Basic approach to veterinary care. In: Quesenberry KE, Carpenter JW, editors. Ferrets, rabbits and rodents clinical medicine and surgery. 3rd edition. St Louis (MO): Elsevier; 2012. p. 13–26.
10. Johnson-Delaney CA. Disorders of the skin. In: Johnson-Delaney CA, editor. Ferret medicine and surgery. Boca Raton (FL): CRC Press; 2016. p. 325–46.
11. Richardson J, Perpinan D. Disorders of the respiratory system. In: Johnson-Delaney CA, editor. Ferret medicine and surgery. Boca Raton (FL): CRC Press; 2016. p. 311–24.
12. Bonami F, Rudd PA, von Messling V. Disease duration determines canine distemper virus neurovirulence. J Virol 2007;81:12066–70.
13. Zehnder AM, Hawkins MG, Kiski MA, et al. An unusual presentation of canine distemper virus infection in a domestic ferret (Mustela putorius furo). Vet Dermatol 2008;19(4):232–8.
14. Stephensen CB, Welter J, Subhashchandra R, et al. Canine Distemper Virus (CDV) infection of ferrets as a model for testing Morbillivirus vaccine strategies: NYVAC- and ALVAC-based CDV recombinants protect against symptomatic infection. J Virol 1997;71(2):1506–13. Available at: https://www.ncbi.nlm.nih.gov/pmc/articles/PMC191207/pdf/711506.pdf. Accessed May 1, 2017.
15. Taylor J, Tartagia J, Riviere M, et al. Applications of canarypox (ALVAC) vectors in human and veterinary vaccination. Dev Biol Stand 1994;82:131–5.
16. Extralabel drug use and AMDUCA: FAQ. Available at: https://www.avma.org/KB/Resources/FAQs/Pages/ELDU-and-AMDUCA-FAQs.aspx. Accessed May 1, 2017.
17. AFA ferret vaccination policy. 2013. Available at: http://www.ferret.org/pdfs/VaccinationPolicy-8-06.pdf. Accessed May 1, 2017.
18. AFA position statement on canine distemper vaccination and titer testing. 2013. Available at: http://www.ferret.org/pdfs/policy_cdv.pdf. Accessed May 1, 2017.
19. Appel MJ, Harris WV. Antibody titers in domestic ferret jills and their kits to canine distemper virus vaccine. J Am Vet Med Assoc 1988;193:323–33.
20. Heller R. AFA distemper titer study. American Ferret Report 2012;21(2):10–1. Available at: http://www.ferret.org/pdfs/health/TiterStudy.pdf. Accessed May 1, 2017.
21. Wagner RA, Bhardwaj N. Serum-neutralizing antibody responses to canine distemper virus vaccines in domestic ferrets (Mustela putorius furo). J Exot Pet Med 2012;21(3):243–7.
22. Pavlacik L, Celer V, Kajerova V, et al. Monitoring of antibodies titre against canine distemper virus in ferrets vaccinated with a live modified vaccine. Acta Vet Brno

2007;76:423–9. Available at: https://actavet.vfu.cz/media/pdf/avb_20070760 30423.pdf. Accessed May 1, 2017.

23. Brown S. Canine distemper in ferrets. 2006. Available at: http://www. veterinarypartner.com/Content.plx?A=674. Accessed May 1, 2017.

24. Niezgoda M, Briggs DJ, Shaddock J, et al. Pathogenesis of experimentally induced rabies in domestic ferrets. Am J Vet Res 1997;58(11):1327–31.

25. Fedaku M. Latency and aborted rabies. In: Baer GM, editor. The natural history of rabies. 2nd edition. Boca Raton (FL): CRC Press; 1991. p. 191–8.

26. Hamir AN, Niezgoda M, Rupprecht CE. Recovery from and clearance of rabies virus in a domestic ferret. J Am Assoc Lab Anim Sci 2011;50(2):248–51. Available at: https://www.ncbi.nlm.nih.gov/pmc/articles/PMC3061427/pdf/jaalas2011000 248.pdf. Accessed May 1, 2017.

27. Brown CM, Slavinski S, Ettestad P, et al. Compendium of animal rabies prevention and control. J Am Vet Med Assoc 2016;248(5):505–17. Available at: http:// nasphv.org/Documents/NASPHVRabiesCompendium.pdf. Accessed May 1, 2017.

28. Rabies: domestic animals. CDC. Available at: https://www.cdc.gov/rabies/ exposure/animals/domestic.html. Accessed May 1, 2017.

29. Rabies Vaccination Certificate. National Association of State Public Health Veterinarians. Available at: http://www.nasphv.org/Documents/RabiesVacCert.pdf. Accessed May 1, 2017.

30. Zoetis defensor press release. Available at: https://www.zoetisus.com/news-and-media/zoetis-defensor-vaccines-now-available-to-help-protect-ferrets-from-rabies.aspx. Accessed May 1, 2017.

31. Rupprecht CE, Gilbert J, Pitts R, et al. Evaluation of an inactivated rabies virus vaccine in domestic ferrets. J Am Vet Med Assoc 1990;196(10):1614–6.

32. Greenacre C. Incidence of adverse events in ferrets vaccinated with distemper or rabies vaccine: 143 cases (1995-2001). J Am Vet Med Assoc 2003;223(5):663–5.

33. Moore GE, Glickman NW, Ward MP, et al. Incidence of and risk factors for adverse events associated with distemper and rabies vaccine administration in ferrets. J Am Vet Med Assoc 2005;226(6):909–12.

34. Murray J. Vaccine injection-site sarcoma in a ferret. J Am Vet Med Assoc 1998; 213(7):955.

35. Munday JS, Stedman NL, Richey LJ. Histology and immunohistochemistry of seven ferret vaccination-site fibrosarcomas. Vet Pathol 2003;40:288–93. Available at: http://journals.sagepub.com/doi/pdf/10.1354/vp.40-3-288. Accessed May 1, 2017.

36. Lewington JH. Ferret husbandry, medicine and surgery. Edinburgh (UK): Butterworth-Heinemann; 2000. p. 289.

37. Roach C. Ferret vaccination-one tenth will do! Advances in exotic, zoo and wild animal medicine. Proceedings of Conference from the Zoological Society of London 2004;113.

38. Von Messling V. The ferret in Morbillivirus research. Biology and diseases of the ferret. 3rd edition. Ames (IA): John Wiley & Sons; 2014. p. 641–51.

39. Da Fontoura Budaszewski R, Hudacek A, Sawatsky B, et al. Inactivated recombinant rabies viruses displaying canine distemper virus glycoproteins induce protective immunity against both pathogens. J Virol 2017;91(8) [pii:e02077–16].

Medication for Behavior Modification in Birds

Yvonne van Zeeland, DVM, MVR, PhD, DECZM (Avian, Small mammal), CPBC

KEYWORDS

- Psittaciformes • Psychoactive drugs • Benzodiazepines • Tricyclic antidepressants
- Serotonin reuptake inhibitors • Dopamine antagonists • Opioid antagonists
- Hormone therapy

KEY POINTS

- Behavior modification therapy and provision of an appropriate living environment are key elements of management of problem behaviors in parrots.
- The use of behavior modifying drugs can be considered adjunct therapy under specific circumstances but only once a proper diagnosis has been established.
- Various classes of behavior modifying drugs exist. To enable selection of the most appropriate drug to use in an individual bird, a thorough diagnostic work-up is needed.
- Due to lack of information on safety and efficacy, psychoactive drugs should be used with caution and gradually titrated to effect.
- When available, therapeutic drug monitoring helps guide therapy, aiming to identify the most appropriate dose and resulting in the least number of side-effects.

INTRODUCTION

Pharmacologic intervention with psychoactive or psychotropic drugs has been long-standing practice in human medicine to treat a variety of mental health issues (eg, schizophrenia, depression, bipolar disorder, and generalized anxiety disorder). Similarly, in veterinary medicine, these drugs have been used with increasing frequency to manage problem behaviors, such as anxiety, aggression, and compulsive behaviors. In addition to psychoactive drugs, hormones, antihistamines, analgesics, and anticonvulsant drugs are also used to alleviate behavior problems that are associated with increased levels of sex hormones, allergies, pain, and/or neurologic dysfunction (eg, epilepsy), respectively. When applied correctly, medication can aid in the treatment of abnormal pathologic behaviors (eg, stereotypic behaviors or those that lack impulse control), help stabilize a patient's emotional state (eg, in case of fear, anxiety, aggression, or hormonal imbalances), and improve its receptiveness to a behavior modification plan, thereby increasing the chances of a successful outcome.

Disclosure Statement: The author has nothing to disclose.
Division of Zoological Medicine, Department of Clinical Sciences of Companion Animals, Faculty of Veterinary Medicine, Utrecht University, Yalelaan 108, Utrecht 3584 CM, The Netherlands
E-mail address: Y.R.A.vanZeeland@uu.nl

Without proper diagnosis of the problem and adequate knowledge of behavior modification drugs (including their mechanism of action, appropriate uses, side effects, and interactions with other medications), however, veterinarians are likely to select an inappropriate drug or implement it incorrectly, which not only poses a risk of therapeutic failure but also can seriously harm a patient because of unintended drug interactions or side effects. Therefore, this article, aims to provide guidelines to the veterinary practitioner in the circumstances in which behavior modification drugs can or cannot be applied as well as provide an overview of the various medications currently used in the pharmacologic management of behavior problems in birds.

BEHAVIOR PROBLEMS: WHEN TO PRESCRIBE AND WHEN NOT TO PRESCRIBE MEDICATION

Just like dogs and cats, parrots and other pet birds can exhibit problem behaviors that can be frustrating for owners and veterinarians to deal with. Some of the more common complaints concern aggression and biting, excessive vocalization (screaming), and feather-damaging and/or self-injurious behavior (**Figs. 1** and **2**).[1] In addition,

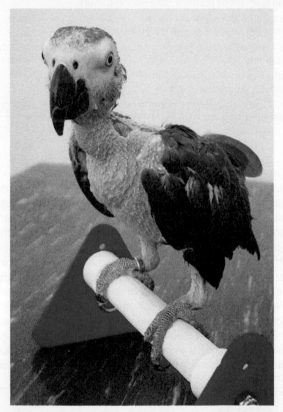

Fig. 1. Feather-damaging behavior (FDB), also referred to as feather-destructive behavior, feather plucking, feather picking, or pterotillomania, is one of the more common behavior problems seen in practice. Underlying causes can vary greatly for each individual case. Often a multifactorial origin is reported, in which various medical, genetic, psychological, neurobiologic, and socioenvironmental factors may play a role. (*Courtesy of* Nico Schoemaker, DVM, PhD, DECZM, DABVP-Avian, Utrecht University, Utrecht, The Netherlands; Yvonne van Zeeland, DVM, MVR, PhD, DECZM, CPBC, Utrecht University, Utrecht, The Netherlands.)

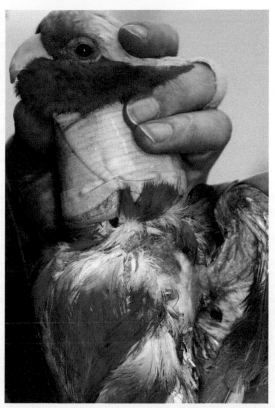

Fig. 2. Aside from feather-damaging behavior, self-injurious behaviors are also commonly seen in psittacine birds. Often times, the self-mutilation is localized to a specific area, whereby the favored area can differ according to the species involved. Cockatoos, for example, often present with severe self-mutilation of feathers, skin, and muscles of the breast, axilla, or patagium (as seen in this galah parrot), whereas Amazon parrots seem to primarily traumatize the feet and legs, and lovebirds predominantly injure themselves in the patagium, neck, axillary region, and back. (*Courtesy of* Nico Schoemaker, DVM, PhD, DECZM, DABVP-Avian, Utrecht University, Utrecht, The Netherlands; Yvonne van Zeeland, DVM, MVR, PhD, DECZM, CPBC, Utrecht University, Utrecht, The Netherlands.)

stereotypic behaviors, anxiety-related disorders (fears and phobias), destructive behaviors, and inappropriate sexual behaviors (eg, excessive egg laying, masturbating, and regurgitation) can be encountered. In many cases, these problem behaviors can be traced back to shortcomings in a bird's living environment or early life history, or represent normal behavior that is misinterpreted or misunderstood by a bird's caregiver (**Box 1**). Moreover, many of the problem behaviors can become exacerbated due to inadvertent reinforcement by 1 or more of the family members. For example, in an attempt to distract a bird that is feather damaging, an owner may worsen the behavior as the bird learns that it will receive attention when it is plucking its feathers. Especially in these situations, where the behavior is the resultant of an attempt of a bird to cope with an inappropriate environment (so-called maladaptive behavior)[15] or in which ignorance or unawareness of an owner plays a part, treatment should first and foremost focus on addressing these underlying issue(s) instead of initiating medical treatment.

Box 1
Common behavior problems in psittacine birds, including their origin and some appropriate interventions

- Destructive behaviors, including chewing, shredding, and stripping of furniture, books, telephone cords, plants, wallpaper, or woodwork, often arise if appropriate chewing substrates and toys are lacking, especially in birds in which the instinctive need to chew is strong (eg, cockatoos and macaws). Provision of appropriate shredding or shredding materials and chewing toys (preferably combined with food to both provide an additional reward and stimulate natural foraging/feeding behavior) as well as supervision of the bird when outside of the cage often help combat these behaviors.

- In the wild, parrots vocalize loudly to keep in touch with the other flock members when leaving to the foraging grounds at dawn and repeat this pattern in the evening when they return to their roosting sites.[2,3] Although attempts can be made to minimize these vocalizations (eg, by darkening the room where the bird is placed in, covering the cage, or providing food or toys as distraction to the bird before the screaming starts), it often is difficult to completely eliminate this behavior. Owners should thus be made aware that these vocalizations are part of the normal behavioral repertoire of a parrot. Similarly, the vocalizations may have had a primary function as a contact call to identify the whereabouts of the family members or gain attention but over time have become excessively loud due to inadvertent reinforcement by 1 or more family members. In those situations, rather than trying to medicate the bird to quiet it down, owners should be made aware of their role in the exacerbation of the problem and provided with advice on how to manage the situation (eg, responding to appropriate calls, providing effective time outs, prevent reinforcement of screaming, and providing other activities that keep the bird preoccupied such as foraging).

- Abnormal repetitive behaviors, such as feather-damaging and stereotypic behaviors, often find their origin in a suboptimal design of the living environment.[4–8] Especially when the bird is unable to perform species-typical behaviors for which it is highly motivated, onset of abnormal repetitive behaviors is likely to occur because of the frustration being redirected (eg, lack of foraging opportunities or allopreening resulting in redirection of this motivation to the bird's plumage) or displaced (eg, feather-damaging behavior occurring in response to exposure of an aversive stimulus). Rather than trying to solve these problem behaviors with medical therapy, these cases benefit the most from a thorough assessment and appropriate management of the bird's living environment.[4,5,9,10] Only in those cases where the bird appears refractory to the husbandry changes that have been made should medical intervention be considered.

- Fear is a common underlying motivation for biting and aggression in prey species, such as parrots. In addition to resorting to biting in an attempt to defend itself (fear biting), a parrot may also bite to protect its territory (territorial aggression) or to protect a person or other bird that is considered its partner (mate-related aggression).[11] Similar to other problem behaviors, positive outcomes of the behavior (eg, retrieving of a hand) can reinforce the behavior (conditioned aggression).[11] The history often reveals the biting to occur only under certain circumstances, for example, in a specific location, such as the cage, or when a specific person is in the vicinity of the bird. Based on the situations under which the biting is occurring, inferences can be made on the underlying motivation, after which recommendations can be made to reduce the biting (eg, use of a 2-enclosure system to reduce territorial aggression, ensuring appropriate bond formation to minimize mate-related aggression).

- Fear is seen in response to a perceived threat in the immediate environment and often results in a classic fight, fright, or flight response. Initially, most birds try to escape and/or avoid the aversive stimulus, but if escape is not possible, fear-biting may result. Over time, classical conditioning (ie, a neutral stimulus becomes aversive through pairing with an aversive stimulus) and operant conditioning (ie, negative reinforcement of the behavior due to removal of the threatening stimulus) can intensify the fear response shown by the bird.[12] In general, fearful behavior can be alleviated by systematic desensitization (ie, reduction or elimination of the fear response by graduated exposure to the aversive stimulus), counterconditioning (ie, pairing the aversive stimulus with a pleasant stimulus to replace the fear with a more pleasant emotion), and response substitution (ie, replacing the fearful behavior with a different, more desirable behavior).[12,13] Generalized anxiety and phobias, however, are often related to poor socialization or traumatic experiences and can be more difficult and time-consuming to treat.[13] To maximize the changes for success, correct identification and control of the aversive stimulus are essential.[13] Moreover, owners need to be able to recognize subtle signs of fear to be able to successfully implement desensitization and counter-conditioning strategies.[13] Use of medication can be considered an adjunct to behavior modification therapy but only if medication can be administered without causing additional stress or fear.

- Inappropriate sexual behaviors (eg, courtship feeding and copulation) often arise due to triggering of the hypothalamus-pituitary-gonadal axis by cues received from the environment, for example, pair bonding stimulated by excessive cuddling and stimulation of the caudal back by the owner, offering of high-caloric diets, and/or provision of nesting materials and an appropriate nesting site.[14] Although hormonal intervention can be used to help alleviate these behaviors, long-term control of these behaviors requires modification of a bird's living environment and ensuring a more appropriate bond formation between owner and the bird.[10,14]

The major reasons the author recommends a reserved approach toward medication in the initial phases of a behavior modification plan are as follows:

- Several studies in humans have shown cognitive behavior therapies (eg, relaxation techniques, mental distractions, or finding of substitute activities to help control addictions) at least equally (if not more) effective than medical treatment, especially in the long term.[16–21] Similar effects are likely to be expected in parrots and other animals.
- Although psychoactive drugs can induce positive changes in the behavior of a patient, they generally only blunt or mask the resulting behavior without addressing the underlying processes or environmental factors that contribute to the behavior problem.
- When adding medication to the treatment regimen, owners may easily perceive this as the mainstay of the therapy and rely on the drugs to deliver a quick fix to the problem. This in turn might affect clients' compliance with the remainder of the treatment plan because they may be less inclined to make the necessary changes in the living environment and/or change their approach to the bird. This likely results in treatment failure and disappointment of an owner.
- Success of behavior therapy and training is highly dependent on adequate memory and learning, which can be negatively influenced by certain psychoactive drugs (especially benzodiazepines [BZPs][22–25]), thus requiring veterinarians to be cautious when administering medication that can potentially affect these processes.
- In various patients, administering the medication can pose challenges because owners are not able to adequately handle a bird or because the handling and medication cause additional stress and anxiety in an already anxious bird, thereby potentially worsening the problem.
- Like any drug, behavior modification drugs can lead to side effects that can be detrimental to a patient.

Thus, rather than starting with medication, a series of interventions should be initiated that aim to educate owners (including the management of their expectations), optimize a bird's living conditions (including elimination of any potential inciting causes), and modify a bird's behavior through implementation of behavior modification strategies (see **Box 1**).[10]

In many patients, environmental management and behavior modification alone allow a problem behavior to be adequately addressed. Nevertheless, some patients may show lack of or insufficient response to these interventions, thereby warranting drugs to be considered an addition to the treatment regimen. This predominantly includes birds with problem behaviors (especially abnormal repetitive behaviors) that have been ongoing for longer periods of time (thereby allowing these to become ritualized)[26] or birds in which the problem behavior can be linked to traumatic events or poor socialization in the past. In these birds, the problem behavior (even though it may have been initiated by an abnormal environment) is suspected to be associated with an abnormal psychology, brain development, or neurochemistry (so-called malfunctional behavior).[15,27] Aside from this group, the use of behavior modifying drugs can also be considered in situations when an (aversive) stimulus cannot be controlled or avoided or when a bird shows overwhelming fear, anxiety, or aggression.

In all these situations, the main goal of the addition of drugs is to increase a bird's receptiveness to the behavioral interventions and changes of the environment. In particular, medications, such as tricyclic antidepressants (TCAs) and selective serotonin reuptake inhibitors (SSRIs), which mediate and modulate the stress-induced block of long-term potentiation (ie, a persistent increase in synaptic strength that underlies the processes of memory and learning),[28] can facilitate implementation of a behavioral and environmental modification plan.[29] As such, behavior modification drugs can also help a bird to improve faster, thereby increasing client satisfaction and motivation to continue the behavior modification plan. Thus, even in patients in which the medication is not an essential part of the treatment regimen, behavior modification drugs may prove a valuable addition as long as they are used appropriately.

DIAGNOSTIC WORK-UP ESSENTIALS — ESTABLISHING A (DIFFERENTIAL) DIAGNOSIS AND RATIONALE FOR THE USE OF BEHAVIOR MODIFICATION DRUGS

Accurate diagnosis and classification of the behavior problem are essential to establishing a behavior modification plan and determine whether a patient could benefit from adding behavior modification drugs to the treatment regimen. Unlike human psychiatry, in which much attention has been paid to diagnosis and classification of psychiatric and behavioral disorders (eg, the *Diagnostic and Statistical Manual of Mental Disorders* [Fifth Edition][30]), clearly structured diagnostic systems to help classify behavioral disorders in animals are not well established in veterinary medicine. Nevertheless, although classification systems clearly have their benefits (eg, facilitating communication between practitioners and behaviorists, allowing comparison of outcomes of different trials, and establishing of ready-to-use protocols for intervention), they are not necessarily the solution to everything. Even in human psychiatry, therapeutic efficacy is seen in only 60% of patients who were provided a treatment that matched their specific diagnosis,[31] emphasizing that accurate diagnosis at most provides clues to develop effective therapeutic strategies. This is because classifications and labeling also have inherent limitations, the primary being that diagnoses are mere phenotypic labels that are unable to capture the entireness of the complex processes that underlie the observed behavioral signs.[32] For example, by labeling a bird "hormonal" or "phobic," it is impossible or at least difficult to formulate specific behavioral modifications, whereas this becomes much easier when the behavior, including the situation in which it occurs, is described in more objective terms (eg, hormonal = a bird lunges toward a person and bites when that person is sitting next to the caregiver while the bird is sitting on the caregiver's lap, or phobic = a bird is making high-pitched vocalizations, flapping its wings, and falls down the perch once someone is approaching it with a large object).

The obvious limitations when dealing with animals instead of human patients do not exempt clinicians from performing a sound diagnostic work-up to try and establish a tentative working diagnosis or list of differential diagnoses that form the basis of a behavior modification plan. This diagnostic-work-up relies on 3 important sources of information:

1. The history of the bird, including a detailed description of the bird's behavior by the owner
2. Direct observations of the bird's behavior by the clinician
3. The physical examination, including any additional diagnostic testing

Based on the findings during these steps, some initial hypotheses can be generated about the underlying motivations and factors contributing to the behavior problem. The antecedent-behavior-consequence method as used by applied behaviorists, in particular, is considered useful in this process (for reviews, see eg, Friedman[33] and van Zeeland and colleagues[10]).

Aside from helping to generate hypotheses about underlying causes, the steps also help establish a rationale for behavioral and medical intervention (ie, whether and which interventions and drugs would be most beneficial to a patient).[34] For example, observation of escape and avoidance behaviors (eg, a bird is trying to retreat from a presented stimulus, such as a hand or object by moving backwards or flying away) provides an indication for anxiety as an underlying motivation (thereby likely requiring desensitization and counter-conditioning strategies with or without anxiolytics), whereas a history or observation of regurgitation, rubbing of the cloaca against objects or nest building behaviors hint toward a potential role for hormones in the problem behavior (which are more likely to benefit from environmental changes and hormone therapy to derail the sexually oriented behavior). Likewise, scratching, wing flapping, and/or sudden, fast, and vigorous biting of the skin or feathers may hint toward pain, irritation, or itch that requires further work-up and treatment of potential underlying medical causes, including the use of drugs such as antihistamines or analgesics.

History

Owners should be thoroughly questioned about their bird's problem behavior, during which the following aspects should be taken into consideration:

- Phenomenology of the behavior (ie, exact description of the behavior displayed by a bird that the owner considered a problem)
- Frequency with which the problem behavior occurs (including its duration)
- Environmental circumstances under which the behavior occurs
- Responses of the owner and other family members after the behavior
- Time of onset of the problem behavior, including age of the bird at that time
- Changes in pattern, frequency, intensity, or duration of the problem behavior over time
- Previous corrective measures or treatments that have been initiated to alleviate the problem behavior, including their effects

Besides questions about the behavioral problem(s), questions should also be asked about a bird's overall behavior, including its relationship and responses to family members and strangers, new situations, and other types of stimuli. Similarly, a parrot's background (eg, rearing history and origin) and current living conditions, including its nutrition, physical, and social environment, daily routine, and preferred enrichments and activities, should be thoroughly evaluated.

Direct Behavioral Observations

A behavioral assessment can either be made by direct observation of a bird's behavior in the clinic or indirectly using recordings of the bird's behavior at home. Direct observations are preferably made at the beginning of a visit or shortly after or during the history taking to prevent significant alterations due to stress from handling.[35,36] It should be emphasized, however, that a bird's behavior in the clinic may be significantly altered by, for example, the presence of an (unfamiliar) observer, a new location, and/or transport to the clinic. To exclude potential influence of these external factors on the bird's behavior, video recordings made by the owner in the home environment often, therefore, provide a helpful addition to complement the direct observations in the clinic.

Aside from observing the bird's behavior in the examination room, it is also important to observe the owner's responses to the bird's behavior (because this may uncover unintended reinforcement of the problem behavior by the owner) as well as the bird's responses to environmental stimuli that are offered as a distraction when performing the problem behavior. If a bird appears to be fixated on a problem behavior and is hardly or not at all distracted by external stimuli, this could either indicate established, hard-to-reverse stereotyped behavior[37] or presence of a strong (internal) stimulus or motivation for the behavior, which is more likely to require medical intervention (eg, using antipsychotics, TCAs, or SSRIs that influence obsessive compulsive behaviors). Similarly, behavior change is more likely difficult to accomplish and to require medical intervention in birds that show either an overwhelming response (eg, fear or aggression) or a total lack of interest in the stimuli they are presented with or are seemingly difficult to engage in activities, such as playing with enrichments (particularly in the home situation).[34,38]

Physical Examination and Ancillary Tests

A full physical examination, consisting of an observation of the patient from a distance, followed by a hands-on examination, is performed to detect physical abnormalities indicative of an underlying disease process that may cause or contribute to the behavioral signs and warrants further diagnostic work-up (eg, blood biochemistry and hematology or imaging) to be performed. Similarly, a further work-up can be indicated in patients in which medical intervention is considered, because certain drugs are contraindicated or may require adjustment of the dosing regimen in case concurrent medical conditions are present. For example, caution is warranted when administering drugs to geriatric patients or those suffering from metabolic, liver, renal, or cardiac diseases.[32] Moreover, because most drugs are metabolized through the hepatic and renal pathways, establishing baseline values is considered essential for monitoring potential side effects.[32] In addition, some medications (eg, SSRIs) are reported to have cardiac side effects,[39] thereby recommending baseline ECGs, especially in patients that have a history of cardiac disease and those that might need sedation or anesthesia.[32]

CHOOSING THE APPROPRIATE DRUG — CONSIDERATIONS FOR DRUG SELECTION

Selection of the appropriate drugs to use for a specific patient necessitates an accurate diagnosis of the behavioral problem of the patient as well as knowledge of drug efficacy and safety (**Box 2**). Veterinarians are, therefore, encouraged to familiarize

Box 2
Checklist for administering medication for behavior modification in birds
The author recommends veterinarians ask themselves the following questions when considering using pharmacologic intervention for behavior modification and ensuring all these can be answered with yes before initiating treatment.
1. Has a thorough behavioral and medical work-up been performed to identify the potential underlying causes for the problem behavior? Has a working diagnosis or differential diagnoses been established?
2. Have the potential underlying medical issues and environmental stressors been adequately dealt with? Has or will an appropriate behavior modification plan be(en) put into place?
3. Is it possible for the owner to medicate the bird without causing additional stress that may exacerbate the existing problems?
4. Does the drug of choice's mechanism of action correspond with the hypothesized neuropathophysiologic processes that underlie the behavioral problem (eg, reduction of anxiety, compulsiveness, or hormonal influence)?
5. Did the medical work-up reveal no contraindications for use of the medication? If the bird is receiving any other medication, is there no interaction with these drugs that warrants caution or adjustment of the dose?
6. Has the owner been informed properly with regard to effects of the therapy and the potential risks (ie, side effects) of the treatment?
7. Has a proper monitoring and follow-up protocol been set in place (eg, frequency of rechecks, monitoring of plasma concentrations, evaluation for presence of side effects)?

themselves with the indications and contraindications, mechanisms of action, and potential side effects of the various classes of behavior modification drugs (discussed later). In general, drug selection primarily depends on the type of behavior problem that is present, whereby the preferred drug comes from the drug class that is most likely to be effective in treating the behavioral problem but poses the least risk of adverse side effects. Given the drug class, the drug selection subsequently depends on the experience with the drug in the given species, whereby the choice falls on the drug with the best-known efficacy.

Unfortunately, for many of the behavior modifying drugs, the absorption, distribution, metabolism, excretion profiles (ie, pharmacokinetic properties of the drug); dose-response curves (ie, pharmacodynamics properties); and therapeutic indices (ie, safety of the drug) in birds are lacking. Placebo-controlled clinical trials demonstrating the effectiveness of behavior modification drugs in birds are also few in number. As a result, data are often extrapolated from studies on other animals or humans. Species differences, however, may be present, which could result in a lack of efficacy or onset of unexpected adverse events. Thus, starting at a low dose and gradual titration of the drug are recommended to determine the optimal dose for individual patients (ie, the dose at which clinical effects are seen without side effects noted). Should (unexpected) side effects be encountered, adjustment of the dose or switching to a different drug or drug class should be considered. Seeming therapeutic failure, on the other hand, first warrants re-evaluation of the original diagnosis and the conditions of drug use (eg, Has the drug been used sufficiently long for it to exert an effect?) before adjusting, switching, or combining medication.

Aside from the behavioral indication, other factors may also play a role in drug selection. For example, in humans, age, gender, and health status of patients have been shown to significantly affect therapeutic efficacy and safety of certain drugs.[31,40–44] Similar findings are therefore to be expected in birds. A study on pharmacokinetics of paroxetine in gray parrots indicated presence of gender-based differences in plasma concentrations.[45] This emphasizes the need to further study the effects of aforementioned patient parameters on the drug's action. Information from studies in humans and other animals may provide initial clues on whether and how these factors may affect the efficacy and tolerability of a drug in a given situation. Presence of health problems (eg, liver or renal disease and arrhythmias) does not necessarily rule out use of a drug but does warrant extra caution with regard to the used dosage and monitoring of potential side effects.

Other issues related to drug selection pertain to the cost, availability, and ease of administration of the medication. Many of the psychoactive drugs need compounding to enable their use in avian patients. This may pose additional challenges, because the effects of compounding on storage and stability of drugs are largely unknown. Moreover, formulation may significantly alter the absorption (and, therefore, clinical efficacy) of drugs as shown in gray parrots, where a commercial suspension of paroxetine resulted in little to no absorption after oral administration compared with a water-based solution of paroxetine.[45] Similarly, challenges may be encountered with intake of medication because of an owner being unable to administer the drugs and/or the bird resisting medication (eg, due to taste aversion of bitter-tasting drugs [**Fig. 3**]).

PSYCHOACTIVE DRUG CLASSES AND THEIR MODE OF ACTION

Psychoactive drugs typically work by changing or balancing the amount of 1 or more neurotransmitters in the brain. Of the various neurotransmitters that have been identified, the following play a pertinent role in regulation of behavior and behavior problems: acetylcholine, dopamine, endorphins, γ-aminobutyric acid (GABA), glutamate, norepinephrine, and serotonin (**Table 1**). Psychoactive drugs exert their effect on one or more of these neurotransmitters, thereby inducing alterations in mood, perception, consciousness, cognition, and behavior. Historically, behavioral drugs have been classified into 6 categories according to their first clinical application in humans:[31]

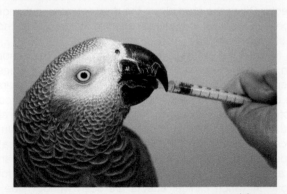

Fig. 3. One of the challenges when attempting behavior modification with drugs is to ensure that the medication is properly administered to the bird. Unfortunately, many owners are not experienced in administering medications to their birds, which can subsequently result in poor therapeutic compliance but also exacerbate an already existent behavior problem (eg, fear or aggression). Operant learning techniques, such as shaping and positive reinforcement, can help teach the birds to voluntarily take in their medication, as demonstrated by this gray parrot (*Psittacus erithacus*). (*Courtesy of* Nico Schoemaker, DVM, PhD, DECZM, DABVP-Avian, Utrecht University, Utrecht, The Netherlands; Yvonne van Zeeland, DVM, MVR, PhD, DECZM, CPBC, Utrecht University, Utrecht, The Netherlands.)

Table 1
Neurotransmitters and their respective functions and associated pathologies

Neurotransmitter	Function	Pathology Resulting from Depletion	Pathology Resulting from Excess
Acetylcholine	Voluntary movement, attention, memory and learning, reward, arousal, and sleep; major neurotransmitter in the autonomic nervous system	Cognitive decline, dementia, Alzheimer disease, myasthenia gravis; blocking of muscarinic receptors results in anticholinergic effects (eg, dry mouth, dry eye, pupillary dilation, tachycardia, constipation, and urinary retention)	Depression
β-Endorphin	Pain relief, feelings of pleasure and contentment	Pain, addiction	Depersonalization disorder, catalepsy
Dopamine	Coordination of motor activities, attention, and learning; modulation of mood (D_1–D_4 receptors), pleasures related to motivation	Behavioral quieting, depression, extrapyramidal motor symptoms (muscle tremors, tics, motor restlessness, and Parkinson disease)	Compulsive and stereotypical behaviors, schizophrenia (in humans)
Epinephrine	Affects sleep, mood, memory and learning, focus and alertness; fight-or-flight response		Fear, agitation; sympathetic effects, leading to, for example, vasoconstriction (α-adrenergic receptors) or vasodilation β_2-adrenergic receptors), increased cardiac contractility (α-adrenergic and β_1-adrenergic receptors), bronchodilation and/or changes in gastrointestinal tract motility (intestinal relaxation, contraction of bladder, and intestinal sphincters)
GABA	Inhibition of excitation and anxiety, behavioral quieting	Seizure activity, Parkinson disease, fear, and phobias	Sleepiness, drowsiness

(continued on next page)

Table 1 (*continued*)			
Neurotransmitter	**Function**	**Pathology Resulting from Depletion**	**Pathology Resulting from Excess**
Glutamate	Excitation; cognitive functions, such as memory and learning	Insomnia, problems with concentration, mental exhaustion, energy depletion	Seizure activity; hyperalgesia; neurodegenerative diseases, such as amyotrophic lateral sclerosis, Parkinson disease, Alzheimer disease
Histamine	Sleep-wake cycle, appetite, sexual behavior, temperature, nociception, gastric acid release, vasodilation, bronchoconstriction, secretory functions (eg, nasal mucous membranes); involved in cognition (memory loss)		Hypersensitivity response, anaphylactic shock
Norepinephrine	Affects mood, functional reward systems, sleep patterns, focus, and arousal/alertness	Depression	Schizophrenia, mania, sympathomimetic effects
Serotonin	Modulation of sleep-wake cycle, temperature, appetite, mood (emotional response), sexual behavior, memory and learning, and impulse control (particularly through serotonin binding to serotonin 1 receptors); also involved in regulation of cardiovascular and endocrine function	Depression, anxiety, irritability, aggression, impulse control and obsessive-compulsive disorders	Agitation, irritability, tremors, hyperreflexia, hyperthermia, sweating, dilated pupils, and diarrhea

1. Anxiolytics, which are primarily used to treat anxiety and anxiety-related disorders
2. Antidepressants, which are used to treat clinical depression as well as some other disorders (eg, anxiety disorders, obsessive compulsive disorders, impulse control disorders, and chronic or neuropathic pain)
3. Antipsychotics, which are predominantly used to treat psychotic symptoms (such as seen in schizophrenia or mania) but also can be used as adjunct therapy to relieve clinical depression

4. Mood stabilizers, which are used to facilitate mood regulation in people experiencing intense, repeated shifts in their mood, as can be seen with bipolar disorder and schizoaffective disorder
5. Stimulants, which are used to help regulate disorganized thought processes and are as such used in the treatment of attention deficit hyperactivity disorder; they furthermore have sympathomimetic activity and increase bodily activity and are therefore also used to treat narcolepsy and for weight reduction.
6. Depressants, which include all hypnotics, sedatives, and anesthetics. This group also includes the opioid antagonists, which can help to overcome endorphin-related or opioid-related addictions by blocking their euphoric effects.

The aforementioned classification is based mainly on a drug's initial clinical application in humans and does not necessarily imply similar functionality in animals. For example, some of the drugs that have traditionally been used as antidepressants in humans have also been found to exert significant anxiolytic effects in animals.[46]

Aside from the classification based on clinical use, drugs are also classified according to their chemical structure and neurochemical activity, whereby drugs in the same category share a similar mechanism of action and side effects.

In veterinary medicine, the most commonly used psychoactive medications include drugs from the antidepressant (ie, TCAs and SSRIs) and anxiolytic (ie, BZPs and azapirones) classes. Of these, however, only 3 have been specifically licensed for use in animals, that is,:

- Fluoxetine (Reconcile), which is licensed for the treatment of dogs with separation anxiety when used in combination with behavior modification
- Clomipramine (Clomicalm), which is also licensed for treatment of separation anxiety in dogs when used in combination with behavior modification
- Selegiline (Anipryl), which is licensed to treat dogs suffering from behavioral problems with an emotional underlying origin

Other uses of these drugs, including the use in other species as well as use of other psychoactive agents, constitutes extralabel use that in the United States falls under the Animal Medicinal Drug Use Clarification Act of 1994. This act requires presence of a valid client-patient-veterinarian relationship as well as an established diagnosis (based on a complete medical and behavioral evaluation) and sound scientific rationale for prescribing the drug made by the veterinarian prescribing the drug (discussed later). If and when a veterinarian feels uncomfortable or insecure about his/her ability to comply with these guidelines, referral of the case to a specialist in behavioral medicine is advised.

In birds, the following classes of psychoactive drugs have been used (**Table 2**):

1. BZPs (eg, diazepam and lorazepam)[47–49]
2. Azapirones (eg, buspirone)[50]
3. TCAs (eg, amitriptyline, clomipramine, and doxepin)[51–56]
4. SSRIs (eg, paroxetine and fluoxetine)[45,51,55,57–62]
5. (Typical) antipsychotics or neuroleptics, which include the phenothiazine derivatives (eg, chlorpromazine),[49] and butyrophenones (eg, haloperidol)[63–65]
6. Opioid antagonists (eg, naltrexone and naloxone)[66,67]

Benzodiazepines

BZPs (eg, diazepam, midazolam, lorazepam, alprazolam, oxazepam, and clorazepate) act by binding to GABA-receptors (primarily $GABA_A$), thereby increasing binding

Table 2
Classes of medications (including mode of action and dosing regimen) that may be considered for behavior modification in birds[a]

Drug Class	Drugs	Mechanism of Action	Indications	Potential Side Effects	Reported Dosing Ranges for Selected Drugs in Birds	Comments
Anticonvulsants	Carbamazepine Gabapentin Levetiracetam Phenobarbital Potassium bromide Zonisamide	Carbamazepine: blocks voltage-gated sodium channels preventing repetitive action potentials Gabapentin: increases synaptic levels of GABA in the CNS Levetiracetam: reduces neurotransmitter release by binding inhibiting presynaptic calcium channels Phenobarbital: potentiates GABA and blocks AMPA-receptor resulting in reduced neuronal excitability Potassium bromide: potentiates the effect of GABA by competing with the transmembrane chloride transport Zonisamide: is thought to block sodium and T-type calcium channels. It has some GABA-ergic activity	Behavior problems arising from seizure activity; potentially beneficial to treat compulsive behaviors (including feather-damaging behavior) and anxiety- or frustration-related aggression, and depression	Mild sedation, lethargy, ataxia, polyuria, polydipsia, polyphagia, anticholinergic effects, bone marrow suppression	Carbamazepine: 3–10 mg/kg q24h; PO, or 166 mg/L drinking water Gabapentin: 10–15 mg/kg q12h PO Levetiracetam: 50–100 mg/kg q8–12h PO Phenobarbital: 1–7 mg/kg q12–24h PO (gray parrots may need dosages of at least 20 mg/kg) Potassium bromide: 25–75 mg/kg Zonisamide: 20–80 mg/kg q12h PO	Can be combined with antipsychotics, such as haloperidol Barbiturates contraindicated in patients with liver disease Carbamazepine contraindicated in patients with renal, hepatic, cardiovascular, or hematologic disorders, including bone marrow suppression Do not combine with antipsychotics or antidepressant; combined use with paroxetine may lower availability of the latter Potassium bromide works synergistically with drugs that have a GABA-ergic effect

Antihistamines	Diphenhydramine, Hydroxyzine	Antihistamine; inverse H$_1$ receptor agonist, thereby blocking effects of histamine	Treatment of allergies; pruritus and pruritus-associated behavioral disorders	Sedation, local anesthesia, antinausea, anticholinergic, antiserotonergic effects	Diphenhydramine: 2–4 mg/kg q12h PO or 2 mg/L drinking water; Hydroxyzine: 2 mg/kg q8-12h; PO, or 30–40 mg/L drinking water	Caution is warranted when using these drugs together with anticholinergic agents or CNS depressants or when using these drugs in patients with hepatic disease
Antipsychotics (neuroleptics)	Chlorpromazine (phenothiaze derivative), Haloperidol (butyrophenone derivative)	Dopamine receptor antagonist	Low-potency antipsychotics (eg, chlorpromazine): mild sedation, tranquilizer; high-potency antipsychotics: treatment of obsessive-compulsive behaviors, including feather-damaging behavior, self-injurious behavior and stereotypic behaviors	Hypotension, bradycardia, decreased seizure threshold, ataxia, sedation, extrapyramidal motor signs, such as muscle tremors and ticks, motor restlessness, agitation and excitability, depression, decreased appetite, regurgitation	Chlorpromazine: 0.1–0.2 mg/kg once; PO, 0.2–1 mL stock solution^b/kg q12–24h; PO, or 1 mL stock solution/120 mL drinking water; Haloperidol: 0.1–0.9 mg/kg q12–24h; PO or 1–2 mg/kg q14–21d; IM	Distinction between typical (eg, chlorpromazine, haloperidol) and atypical antipsychotics (eg, clozapine, risperidone), of which the latter have less side effects. Chlorpromazine is less specific then haloperidol and mainly results in sedation. Low-potency antipsychotics may be combined with BZPs or SSRIs; use with other antipsychotics or TCAs is contraindicated.
Azapirones	Buspirone	Acts as a serotonin agonist	Anxiolytic, treatment of anxiety disorders	A large range of side effects are reported in people ranging from dizziness to gastrointestinal signs, alterations in social behavior, and pruritus. Generally, these are mild and noted soon after initiation of therapy.	Buspirone: 0.5 mg/kg q12h; PO	Combined use with either itraconazole, rifampicin and haloperidol may increase the plasma concentration of buspirone. Carbamazepine, on the other hand decreases plasma concentrations of buspirone.

(continued on next page)

Table 2
(continued)

Drug Class	Drugs	Mechanism of Action	Indications	Potential Side Effects	Reported Dosing Ranges for Selected Drugs in Birds	Comments
BZPs	Diazepam, lorazepam	Binds to GABA$_A$ receptor thereby potentiating the inhibitory effects of GABA	Anticonvulsant; skeletal muscle relaxant; appetite stimulant; short-term management of acute and intermittent behavior problems, in particular those involving fear, anxiety, and phobia, feather picking or aggression. Also useful to facilitate collar placement	Sedation, ataxia, muscle weakness, hyperphagia, disinhibition of aggression, paradoxic excitation, memory deficits (also: inhibition of learning); potentially fatal hepatic necrosis after oral dosing in cats; neutropenia, jaundice, and anemia have been reported after long-term use in humans.	Diazepam: 0.25–1.5 mg/kg q8–24h; IM, 0.5–4 mg/kg q6–24h; PO, or 10–20 mg/L drinking water Lorazepam: 0.1 mg/kg q12h; PO Midazolam: 0.1–2 mg/kg IM or IV, 1–2 mg/kg intranasally	BZPs act as sedatives at low dosages, as anxiolytics at moderate dosages; and as hypnotics at high dosages Risk of drug dependence has been reported in humans, therefore recommending gradual withdrawal after chronic dosing BZPs can be used concurrently with other psychoactive drugs (eg, antipsychotics, TCAs and SSRIs) to help to overcome the delayed efficacy of the other drugs. Concurrent dosing requires lowering of the dose to prevent CNS depression. Avoid in patients with CNS or respiratory depression, obesity, renal or hepatic failure
β-Blockers	Propranolol	Selectively prohibits the reconsolidation of the fear memory	Treatment of anxiety disorders	Bradycardia, lethargy, hypotension, syncope	No dose reported in birds	Has been reported effective for treating anxiety in dogs, but a meta-analysis of its use in humans provided insufficient support for the use of propranolol in the treatment of anxiety disorders

		Indication	Side effects	Dosage	Comments
GnRH agonists	Deslorelin Leuprolide acetate	Down-regulation of GnRH, after initial increase, and thereby LH (and FSH)	Treatment of sexual-related behavior disorders	None reported	Deslorelin: 4.7 and 9.4 mg (slow-release implant); q3–6 mo Leuprolide acetate: 100–800 µg/kg q2–3 wk	A delayed response of up to 2 wk may be seen, due to the initial rise of GnRH Because both GnRH agonists have the same mode of action, deslorelin has a longer duration of action and is also registered for use in animals, there is no reason to still use leuprolide acetate.
Melatonin	Melatonin	Stimulates release of GnIH thereby down-regulating GnRH	Treatment of aggression, undesired sexual related behavior, and anxiety disorders	Mild sedation may occur in dosages >1 mg/kg	0.5–3 mg/kg	Further studies are needed to determine optimal dosage and indication
NSAIDs	Meloxicam Carprofen Piroxicam	Analgesic, anti-inflammatory and antipyretic action through inhibition of prostaglandin synthesis	Treatment of pain-related behaviors	May cause gastrointestinal bleeding and renal failure	Meloxicam: 0.5–1.5 mg/kg q12–24h PO Carprofen: 1–10 mg/kg q12–24h IM Piroxicam: 0.5 mg/kg q12h PO	Only COX-2 specific drugs are mentioned because these have the lowest risk of side effects. Great species variation in dose. For meloxicam: gray parrot 0.5 mg/kg q24h; Amazon parrot 1.5 mg/kg q12h
Opiate receptor antagonists	Naloxone Naltrexone	Block effects of endogenous endorphins	Treatment of stereotypies and other compulsive or self-injurious behavior, including feather-damaging behavior and self-injurious behavior; analgesia	Increased anxiety, gastrointestinal problems, such as abdominal cramps, nausea, vomiting, and constipation	Naloxone: 2 mg/kg; IV Naltrexone: 1.5 mg/kg q8–12h; PO	Is expected to work predominantly in the early phases, when behavior is not ritualized. Reduction in feather-damaging behavior can be observed within 20 min postinjection (for naloxone) Contraindicated in patients with liver disease

(continued on next page)

Table 2
(continued)

Drug Class	Drugs	Mechanism of Action	Indications	Potential Side Effects	Reported Dosing Ranges for Selected Drugs in Birds	Comments
SSRIs	Fluoxetine Paroxetine Zimelidine	Selective block of serotonin reuptake at presynaptic membrane, leading to an increased availability of serotonin; increased sensitivity to serotonin, with secondary down-regulation of postsynaptic receptors	Compulsive and impulsive disorders (including feather-damaging behavior and self-injurious behavior), fear, phobias, and anxiety-related disorders, aggression	Generally mild side effects, including lethargy, sedation, insomnia, loss of appetite, weight loss, nausea, diarrhea, mild ataxia, and potential lowering of seizure threshold; serotonin syndrome can occur on sudden withdrawal from medication.ᶜ In pigeons, the use of an SSRI has been shown to result in a decrease of time spent on rapid-eye-movment sleep.	Fluoxetine: 1–5 mg/kg q24h; PO Paroxetine: 1–4 mg/kg q12–24h; PO Zimelidine: 7.5 mg/kg IM (10 mg/kg may cause regurgitation)	Preferred treatment of affective- and anxiety-related disorders Delayed onset of action of approximately 2–6 wk (clinical effects seen in cats within 1–2 wk) Caution warranted in patients with seizures and altered blood glucose (monitoring of blood glucose is advised) Do not use in combination with MAOIs, TCAs, anticonvulsant drugs, and antipsychotics

TCAs Amitriptyline Clomipramine Doxepin Nortriptyline	Block norepinephrine and serotonin reuptake; act as competitive antagonists at muscarinic acetylcholine, histaminergic H_1, and α_1-adrenergic or α_2-adrenergic receptors	Treatment of fear, phobia, anxiety, and aggression; depression; impulsive and obsessive compulsive disorders (including feather-damaging behavior and self-injurious behavior); alleviation of chronic neuropathic pain; treatment of pruritic conditions (including feather-damaging behavior) due to antihistamine action	Sedation, lethargy, hyperactivity, paradoxic anxiety, agitation, ataxia, seizures, hallucinations, tachycardia, mydriasis, decreased tear production, dry mouth, gastrointestinal upset, regurgitation, constipation, change in appetite, increased thirst, urinary retention	Amitriptyline: 1–5 mg/kg q12–24h; PO; 9 mg/kg may be needed to achieve serum concentrations within the human therapeutic range (although this may be toxic to some birds) Clomipramine: 0.5–9.5 mg/kg q12–24h; PO Doxepin 0.5–5 mg/kg q12–24h; PO Nortriptyline: 16 mg/L drinking water	Clinical effects and improvement generally not seen until 2–4 wk after start of treatment Clomipramine most selective for serotonin reuptake inhibition; doxepin and amitriptyline have strongest antihistamine effects Recommended to start with low dose and gradually titrate to effect; gradual tapering off to minimize risk of withdrawal syndrome Can be combined with anxiolytics (eg, buspirone, BZPs); do not use in combination with MAOIs, antipsychotics, anticholinergics, antidepressants, barbiturates, anticonvulsants, thyroid supplements or antithyroid medication Contraindicated in patients with blood glucose alterations, adrenal disorders, glaucoma, seizures, hepathopathy, or cardiac disease.

Abbreviations: AMPA, α-amino-3-hydroxy-5-methyl-4-isoxazolepropionic acid; IM, intramuscular; IV, intravenous; MAOI, monoamine oxidase inhibitor.

[a] Note: most of the dosages in this table have been derived from case reports and/or anecdotal evidence. Because information on pharmacokinetics, pharmacodynamics, efficacy and toxicity are currently lacking for most of these drugs, no specific recommendations can be made at this stage.

[b] Stock solution: 125-mg chlorpromazine in 31-mL simple syrup.

[c] A potentially fatal condition that is characterized by onset of 1 or more of the following symptoms: diarrhea; restlessness; extreme agitation, hyperreflexia, and autonomic instability with possible rapid fluctuations in vital signs; myoclonus, seizures, hyperthermia, uncontrollable shivering, and rigidity; and delirium, coma, status epilepticus, cardiovascular collapse, and death.

affinity of the receptor for GABA. As a result, these drugs potentiate the inhibitory effects of GABA, whereby their effects are dose dependent: at low dosages, BZPs act as sedatives; at moderate dosages, they act as anxiolytics; and at high dosages, they act as hypnotics, facilitating sleep.[68] Because of their rapid onset of action, BZPs are considered particularly beneficial for short-term treatment of acute and intermittent fear and anxiety-related behaviors (including fear-related aggression). In addition, BZPs can be useful in the treatment of (acute episodes of) fear-related or stress-related feather damaging and self-injurious behaviors. BZPs furthermore have sedative, appetite-stimulating, and anticonvulsant effects (with a rapid onset of action) and, therefore, can also be considered useful in the treatment of acute seizures or anorexia; to facilitate social interaction and in situations where (temporary) sedation may be necessary, for example, to facilitate the acceptance of (Elizabethan) collars by the bird.[38,55,69] For the drugs to be effective, they must generally be given at least an hour before the anticipated stimulus (if administered orally) and at least before the bird starts displaying signs of distress. BZPs can be used in conjunction with other psychoactive drugs (eg, TCAs and SSRIs) to help overcome the period needed for onset of action of these drugs. Main disadvantages include long-term dependence and tolerance, necessitating the dose to be increased.[70] Moreover, BZPs interfere with the ability to learn and thus may negatively affect the outcome of a behavior modification plan (except in situations where formation of aversive associations is preferred [eg, when visiting a veterinarian]). Withdrawal signs may also occur after cessation of treatment.[71]

Azapirones

Azapirones (of which buspirone is the only one commercially available) are serotonin 1A agonists that act as full agonists at the presynaptic serotonin 1A receptors (resulting in decreased serotonin synthesis and inhibition of neuronal firing) and as partial agonists at postsynaptic serotonin 1A receptors.[72,73] In humans, buspirone has been used in the treatment of generalized anxiety disorder and the treatment of aggression associated with impaired social interaction but has been found ineffective for the treatment of panic disorder.[74–76] In animal models, buspirone has also shown efficacy in treatment of conditioned avoidance responses[77] and has anecdotally been used to treat paradoxic anxiety caused by clomipramine.[50] Compared with BZPs, buspirone produces no sedation, no cognitive impairment, and low risk of side effects.[72,73,78] Moreover, it has low abuse potential and low risk of withdrawal concerns, thereby rendering it favorable to BZPs for long-term treatment of anxiety. To evaluate its effect, buspirone needs to be administered for several weeks because no immediate behavioral effects are produced.[72,73]

Tricyclic Antidepressants

TCAs, including amitriptyline, imipramine, clomipramine, nortriptyline, and doxepin, potentiate the effects of biogenic amines (ie, norepinephrine, epinephrine, dopamine, serotonin, and histamine) to varying degrees. TCAs may either block the neurotransmitter reuptake (norepinephrine, serotonin, and — to a lesser extent — dopamine) or act as competitive antagonists at the respective muscarinic acetylcholine, histaminergic H_1, and α_1-adrenergic or α_2-adrenergic receptors (acetylcholine, histamine, and norepinephrine).[79] Therapeutic effects are believed to result primarily from inhibition of norepinephrine and serotonin reuptake, whereas blockage of α-adrenergic, antihistaminic, and anticholinergic activities is believed to account for the various side effects seen after administration of these drugs.[79]

Because TCAs exert their effect (in part) through down-regulation of the receptors, their onset of action is delayed (ie, improvement may not be noticeable until 2–4 weeks after initiation of the treatment).[79]

In humans, TCAs are commonly used to treat depression, panic disorders, phobias, neuropathic pain and obsessive-compulsive behaviors. Clomipramine, in particular, which has the highest selectivity for serotonin reuptake inhibition, is used widely in veterinary medicine for treating compulsive disorders, including feather-damaging behavior.[38,52,54,80,81] Similar to humans, TCAs may also be indicated in the treatment of fear, phobia, anxiety, and aggression or to alleviate chronic neuropathic pain.[38,79] Amitriptyline and doxepin, which produce the strongest antihistaminergic effects, may furthermore be useful to treat pruritus resulting from allergic conditions based on favorable efficacy in birds suspected of an allergy-related form of feather-damaging behavior.[38,53,82]

Because of their anticholinergic, antihistaminergic, and adrenergic effects, TCAs are generally considered to have narrow therapeutic safety, with no specific antidotes available in case of overdosing.[79] Side effects seen after TCA administration in birds include increased wariness, anxiety, agitation, depression, increased appetite, and neurologic signs (including hallucinations, dystonia, ataxia, and tremors).[50,53,55,56,82,83] Many of these side effects were only seen afer administration of higher dosages (ie, >4 mg/kg clomipramine every 12 hours orally; 9 mg/kg amytriptiline orally, single dose).[50,56] In two birds (a green-winged macaw and Moluccan cockatoo), however, severe neurologic signs and death were seen at lower dosages (ie, 3 mg/kg clomipramine every 12 hours orally; 2 mg/kg imipramine every 12 hours orally),[55] emphasizing that caution should be exercised when administering these drugs as species or individuals may respond differently to the treatment. Gradual dose titration and careful, continued monitoring for the presence of side effects are, therefore, recommended when starting a patient on TCAs.

Selective Serotonin Reuptake Inhibitors

SSRIs, including fluoxetine, fluvoxamine, sertraline, paroxetine, and zimelidine, selectively block the reuptake of serotonin into the presynaptic membrane, thereby increasing availability of serotonin. In addition, SSRIs can increase the sensitivity of the postsynaptic receptors to serotonin.[84] SSRIs usually need to be administered for at least 2 weeks to 6 weeks to induce down-regulation of postsynaptic receptors and the associated clinical effects.[84] Common behavioral indications include compulsive and impulsive disorders (including feather-damaging behavior and self-injurious behaviors), fear, phobias, and anxiety-related disorders, and aggression.[38,84] Because of their mood-stabilizing effect, SSRIs are also considered the preferred drugs for treating affective or anxiety-related disorders.

Of the various SSRIs that are available, paroxetine is one of the most potent and selective, thereby posing minimal risk of central and autonomous side effects.[85] Paroxetine has been found beneficial in treating phobias and feather-damaging behavior in birds.[10,38,55,60] Reports concerning its efficacy, however, are sparse and limited to case reports and anecdotal evidence, with no controlled clinical trials available to support these findings. A study in gray parrots demonstrated a dose of 4-mg/kg paroxetine hydrochloride, every12 hours orally, to result in plasma concentrations within the therapeutic range recommended for the treatment of depression in humans.[45] Large interindividual differences were present, however, in plasma concentrations, indicating the need for further clinical trials into its efficacy, whereby therapeutic drug monitoring may potentially help establish the correct dosing regimen for individual patients. In addition to paroxetine, fluoxetine has also been shown promising in birds with feather-damaging behavior and toe-chewing, although relapses were commonly seen.[57,63]

Because of their selectivity, which results in fewer side effects compared with TCAs, SSRIs are considered the safer choice in humans.[86,87] Gradual withdrawal is recommended to prevent serotonin syndrome.[84]

Antipsychotics

Antipsychotics or neuroleptics are classified as low-potency agents (eg, acepromazine and chlorpromazine) and high-potency agents (eg, haloperidol and risperidone). These drugs act as dopamine receptor antagonists, resulting in behavioral quieting or ataraxia (ie, decreased emotional reactivity and relative indifference to stressful situations) and suppression of spontaneous movements without affecting spinal and pain reflexes.[88] In veterinary medicine, low-potency antipsychotics are commonly used as tranquilizers, whereas high-potency antipsychotics have been used to reduce compulsive behaviors in various animal species, including compulsive feather-damaging and self-injurious behaviors in parrots.[63–65,88,89]

Of the high-potency antipsychotics available, haloperidol is the most commonly used. Haloperidol is available as both long-acting injectable and oral formulations. Although the long-acting injectable can be advantageous to use in birds because of reduced dosing frequency and omitting the need for an owner to administer the medication, to the author's knowledge there currently is no information available on the pharmacokinetics of this drug in birds. Due to the greater risks associated with overdosing of long-acting formulations, the author therefore recommends against the use of these in the treatment of avian patients.

Compared with high-potency agents, low-potency antipsychotics generally require larger doses and result in more sedation and greater anticholinergic and cardiovascular effects but have a lower incidence of neurologic side effects (ie, extrapyramidal side effects, including Parkinson-like symptoms, dystonia, dyskinesia, and akathisia).[88] Such neurologic side effects have also been reported in birds.[64,65] Most of these side effects are primarily encountered within the first few days after initiation of treatment, with only few occurring in the long term (ie, after treatment of several months up to years).[63–65] Anecdotally, haloperidol has been reported to result in sudden death in a hyacinth macaw and a red-bellied macaw.[64] Similarly, evidence suggests that Quaker parakeets and cockatoo species may be more sensitive to side effects. Caution and lowering of the dose may thus be warranted in these species.[64] Besides species differences in side effects, conflicting results also have been reported concerning the efficacy of antipsychotic drugs in the treatment of psittacine behavior problems. For example, favorable results were achieved after the use of haloperidol in automutilating cockatoos,[51,64,65] whereas no obvious improvement was seen in others.[63] Thus, further studies into dosing regimen and efficacy (including species differences therein) are needed to enable evidence-based decisions to be made on the use of antipsychotics in birds. It should be remembered, however, that these drugs exert their effect (at least in part) through generalized behavioral quieting because of their sedative effects and, therefore, may not specifically address the underlying neuropathophysiology. This is also the reason why this group of drugs has lost a great deal of its popularity in the veterinary and behavior fields.

Opioid Antagonists

Opioid or narcotic antagonists (eg, naloxone and naltrexone) counteract the effects of endogenous opioids that are released during stress. Endogenous opioids activate the dopaminergic system, induce analgesia, and block pain, which are all factors believed to contribute in the onset of stereotypical and self-injurious behaviors.[90] By reversing the opioid-induced analgesia, opioid antagonists have the potential to block the reinforcing effects of self-injurious behaviors and might, therefore, be useful in the diagnosis and treatment of stereotypic and other compulsive or self-injurious behaviors in zoo and companion animals.[91–95] The suppression of these behaviors, however, may only last for a short while, thereby rendering these drugs primarily beneficial in acute presentations when the behavior is not yet ritualized (ie, shortly after their onset). In parrots, opioid antagonists, such as naltrexone, might be helpful to treat early-stage feather-damaging and self-injurious behaviors, with a positive response seen in more than 75% of treated birds.[67] More than half of these birds, however, wore collars or restraint devices, thereby potentially biasing the outcomes, although in several individuals the collar was removed prior to the end of the trial.

HORMONE THERAPY FOR TREATMENT OF REPRODUCTIVE-RELATED BEHAVIORS

Reproduction-related behaviors (eg, territoriality, aggression toward humans in the house, courtship activity, masturbation, and some forms of feather-damaging behavior) can be seen in birds of both genders during the breeding season. Although reproduction-related behaviors should be considered normal behaviors, they can become a problem when they are directed toward humans or result in medical conditions, such as a cloacal prolapse. Most commonly, birds displaying unwanted reproduction-related behaviors have been reared by humans and lack an avian companion.[96] Measurement of plasma sex steroids and endoscopic evaluation of the gonads can be used to assess the reproductive status of the bird, thereby aiding in the diagnosis.[35,97]

Historically, medroxyprogesterone acetate has been used in the management of reproductive-related conditions in birds. Due to the abundance of side-effects seen with this hormone and with the introduction of other effective therapies, this treatment option has effectively become obsolete.[10] Nowadays, slow-release depot gonadotropin-releasing hormone (GnRH) agonists, such as deslorelin or leuprolide acetate, are the primary drug of choice to be used in patients with suspected reproductive-related behavior problems.[10,96] These depot GnRH agonists have a similar mode of action and result in an initial increase of the gonadotropins, luteinizing hormone (LH) and follicle-stimulating hormone (FSH),[98,99] which is followed within the next weeks with a decrease in gonadotropin production to levels under the detection limit of the assay. It is hypothesized that either a down-regulation of gonadotropin receptors in the pituitary gland occurs or that the release of gonadotropins no longer occurs due to the loss of pulsatile release of GnRH. Before the deslorelin-containing implants came onto the market for use in animals, leuprolide acetate — an injectable depot GnRH-agonist registered for use in humans —was considered the drug of choice. Because slow-release deslorelin implants are registered for use in animals (**Fig. 4**), have a longer duration of action, and do not need off-label storage, however, as is required after dissolving the leuprolide acetate, the use of these implants is favored over the use of leuprolide acetate. Anecdotal reports have shown both drugs to be effective in treatment of reproductive-related behaviors, with leuprolide acetate providing 73% overall improvement, with temporary resolution in 89% of chronic egg-laying psittacines,[100] and deslorelin resulting in an overall improvement of 50% (varying from 34% in case of masturbation to 62% in case of territorial aggression) of birds with reproductive-related behavioral problems.[96] If the environment retains the triggers for reproductive stimulation, however, the problems are likely to recur despite

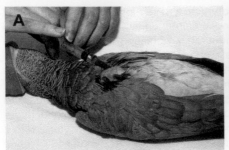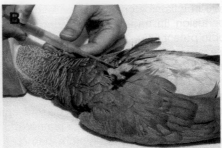

Fig. 4. To reduce reproductive-related behaviors, long-acting depot deslorelin-containing implants can be used. These implants are best placed subcutaneously in between the shoulder blades. To facilitate placement, a small amount of fluid can be injected subcutaneously prior to placement of the implant (*A*). The needle can then be inserted into the fluid bubble to place the implant (*B*). Analgesics (eg lidocaine, bupivacaine) can be added to the fluid for additional pain relief. (*Courtesy of* Nico Schoemaker, DVM, PhD, DECZM, DABVP-Avian, Utrecht University, Utrecht, The Netherlands; Yvonne van Zeeland, DVM, MVR, PhD, DECZM, CPBC, Utrecht University, Utrecht, The Netherlands.)

hormone therapy. Thus, environmental triggers must effectively be dealt with before long-term effects can be achieved.

Recently, a study also reported favorable outcomes after administration of melatonin, with efficacy reported in 3 of 4 birds treated for aggression, 1 of 3 birds treated for undesired hormonal behavior, and 2 of 4 birds treated for anxiety-related behavior problems.[101] Its action is hypothesized to be similar to the depot GnRH-agonists, whereby the melatonin-induced release of gonadotropin-inhibiting hormone (GnIH) down-regulates the synthesis and release of GnRH, thereby inhibiting the synthesis and release of the gonadotropins LH and FSH.[102] In birds with feather-damaging behavior, melatonin yielded no clinical improvement.[101]

THERAPY FOR PAIN-RELATED BEHAVIORS

Any painful condition may initiate a change in behavior, resulting in defensive forms of aggression (biting), feather-damaging, and/or self-injurious behavior. It is, therefore, important to determine under what preceding circumstances the behavior occurs to aid in localizing the origin/location of the pain. The painful area is usually located in the region that is targeted by the bird or the region that evokes a biting response in the bird once it is approached or touched.

When suspecting pain as the underlying cause for the behavior problem(s), a trial with 1 or more analgesics may be warranted. The analgesic effects can particularly be beneficial in patients with self-injurious behaviors that is caused by pain or those that are experiencing pain as a result of the self-injurious behaviors.[38] The drugs' duration of action, however, may be a limiting factor in successful, long-lasting pain relief, because some (eg, butorphanol) need to be given a frequently as 6 times per day. However, sustained release formulations, which have been reported to provide analgesia in Amazon parrots for up to 5 days,[103] may provide a practical solution once they become commercially available.

Different classes of analgesic drugs can be used to prevent, eliminate, or reduce the nociceptive input at different stages, forming the basis of a multimodal approach to pain management.[104] Nonsteroidal anti-inflammatory drugs (NSAIDs) exert their analgesic effects by inhibiting the enzymes cyclooxygenase (COX)-1 and COX-2. The COX enzymes are responsible for the production of prostaglandins, which play an important role in inflammatory processes and in regulating renal and gastrointestinal mucosal perfusion. In addition, they have an antipyretic activity. Meloxicam and carprofen, both potent COX-2 inhibitors, are currently the most frequently used NSAIDs in birds. Because COX-2 inhibitors supposedly have less effect on the gastrointestinal mucosa and kidney function, these drugs are considered safer compared with other NSAIDs.[104]

Opioids are used for the management of moderate to severe pain. They exert their analgesic effects by binding to the opioid receptors. Butorphanol is most commonly used in birds because it has a high affinity for the κ-opioid receptor, which is considered the predominant receptor in birds.[104] TCAs have also been indicated as potential treatment agents to ameliorate chronic neuropathic pain.[38,55]

Gabapentin, a structural analog of the neurotransmitter GABA, has also anecdotally been used in the treatment of (presumed) neuropathic pain in birds.[105–107] Although the mechanism of action of gabapentin is not completely understood, the drug is thought to bind to the α2-δ subunit of voltage-gated calcium channels, thereby decreasing the release of excitatory neurotransmitters.[108] In a recent pharmacokinetic study in Amazon parrots, a dose of 15 mg/kg, every 8 hours, was found to result in therapeutic plasma levels,[8,109] whereas in great horned owls, sufficient plasma concentrations were achieved after giving 11 mg/kg every 8 hours.[110] These dosages are higher than the previously recommended dose of 10 mg/kg every 12 hours[49] and show that the recommended dose may be dependent on the species. Overdosing may result in diarrhea, ataxia, decreased mental alertness, agitation, and hyperesthesia.[111]

THERAPY FOR PRURITUS-ASSOCIATED BEHAVIORS

Similar to pain, pruritus may be at the basis of many self-injurious behaviors, including feather-damaging behavior. This pruritus may be the end result of various types of infections or inflammatory or neoplastic skin diseases. Although hypersensitivity responses have been suspected in avian patients, diagnosis of disease is difficult due to the diminished response of birds to histamine after intradermal testing.[112] As a result, clinicians have to rely on histopathologic results of skin and/or feather follicle biopsy to make a tentative diagnosis of allergic skin disease, while ruling out other causes of pruritus.[113,114]

In cases of a tentative diagnosis of allergic skin disease, treatment should be aimed at eliminating the potential (food and contact) allergens from the bird's environment. This can prove difficult, however. In cases of extreme pruritus, treatment can also be initiated with antihistaminergic drugs (eg, diphenhydramine or hydroxyzine), which block the physiologic effects of histamine by preventing it from binding to the postsynaptic H_1 receptors.[115] The experience with the use of antihistaminergic drugs is limited, however, with only 1 case report reporting successful resolution of feather-damaging behavior and pruritus in a parrot after a combination treatment with hydroxyzine and eicosapentaenoic acid.[116] Other options for alleviation of pruritus and pruritus-associated behaviors include TCAs (amitryptiline and doxepin)[38,53,82] and corticosteroids, although the latter should be used with caution due to their immunosuppressive effects.[117]

THERAPEUTIC OPTIONS IN CASES OF CONVULSIVE BEHAVIORS

Anticonvulsant drugs are not commonly used in behavioral medicine, unless idiopathic epilepsy warrants long-term treatment. When confronted with a parrot with acute seizures, BZPs (eg, diazepam and midazolam) in particular are considered useful because they have an anticonvulsant effect with a rapid onset of action.[118] The duration of action, however, is short and they have a sedative effect. For long-term management of seizure activity, phenobarbital (a drug belonging to the class of barbiturates that enhance the action of GABA) is commonly used.[118] Barbiturate use is contraindicated, however, in patients with hepatic disease and those receiving other central nervous system (CNS) drugs (eg, antipsychotics and/or antidepressants) because concurrent administration of these drugs may result in CNS depression.[119] In addition, combined administration of, for example, paroxetine and phenobarbital, may decrease plasma concentrations of paroxetine, thereby limiting its effects.[120] A study in gray parrots has shown that much higher and frequent dosages are needed to achieve similar plasma concentrations as those found effective in humans.[121] It is, therefore, important to measure plasma concentrations of phenobarbital to evaluate the treatment of any bird with epilepsy.

Carbamazepine is an anticonvulsant drug with mood-stabilizing properties. This drug is, therefore, considered useful in the treatment of humans with depression, mania, and/or explosive aggression. In birds, carbamazepine may likewise be useful to treat compulsive disorders (including feather-damaging behavior) and fear-related or frustration-related aggression.[10] In the treatment of birds with compulsive feather-damaging behavior or self-mutilation, it has been proposed to combine the administration of carbamazepine with chlorpromazine or haloperidol, particularly during the initial first 2 weeks of treatment.[38]

Gabapentin, levetiracetam, and zonisamide have also been proposed as potential anticonvulsant drugs in birds.[118,122–124] The advantage of these drugs is that they are not metabolized in the liver and therefore may be used in birds with hepatic disease. Pharmacokinetic studies have revealed similar findings as with phenobarbital in that higher dosages are needed compared with mammals. Because large variations in plasma concentrations were found with these drugs, individual drug monitoring is recommended during treatment with these drugs.[124]

MONITORING AND FOLLOW-UP

To evaluate whether the treatment has the desired (and no adverse) effects, regular monitoring and follow-up of patients are recommended. Regular contact with the owner is needed to discuss alterations in the behavior, including presence of side effects. To obtain objective, meaningful assessments, owners need to be educated to be observant and recognize signs indicative of potential adverse effects. Moreover, they should be encouraged to immediately contact a clinician if suspecting a problem. Regular rechecks in the clinic are also advised during which a physical examination and laboratory tests may be performed. Whether and which tests to perform depends on the type of drug that is used. For most drugs, evaluation of renal and liver function (ie, annually in younger birds and biannually in older birds) is indicated because alteration of the function of these organs can affect the metabolism and clearance of the drugs, thereby warranting adjustment of the dose.[32] Similarly, ECGs should be considered in patients treated with psychoactive medications with known cardiac side effects (eg, SSRIs and phenothiazines).[32] Ideally, therapeutic drug monitoring is performed by a qualified laboratory because this can help guide the course of action in cases of poor clinical response or observation of side effects. Although some initial studies have been performed into plasma concentrations of specific psychoactive agents (ie, amitriptyline and paroxetine) after single or repeated dosing,[45,56] no studies have yet been performed to link plasma concentrations to clinical effects in birds. As a result, clinicians primarily have to rely on data regarding therapeutic windows established in humans and other species. Species, age, and gender differences may exist, however, emphasizing that adequate clinical response are not always achieved by giving the same dose of the same drug to any patient.

In general, starting at a low dose and gradual titration until a clinical effect or adverse effects are observed is recommended. Unless a patient exhibits adverse effects, treatment should be attempted for at least the time period that is needed for the drugs to take effect (ie, 1 week for BZPs and 1 month for most other drugs [**Box 3**]). If, after this period, insufficient response but no adverse effects are seen, the dose can be gradually increased. Should the maximum dose be reached or adverse effects encountered without the problem behavior adequately resolved, switching to another drug (either one from the same family or one from a different family) can be attempted.

Because combined use of psychoactive drugs can potentially result in undesired interactions, withdrawal of 1 drug before starting the next is generally recommended (although some drugs, such as TCAs and SSRIs, can be combined with BZPs to obtain faster results). For example, in humans, the recommended drug-free time for SSRIs is 2 weeks (ie, at least 2 drug-free dosing intervals or 2+ half-lives—the general rule of thumb for withdrawal of any drug).[32] Rather than stopping abruptly, drugs should be weaned to minimize the risk of withdrawal symptoms as well as enable determination of the least effective dose (should long-term maintenance therapy be required). Gradual tapering of the dose is generally accomplished over the same period of time as needed for the onset of clinical effect, or more slower (if possible). Weaning can generally be done rapidly (ie, a reduction of the total daily dose by 25% every week) in patients with minor problems and a rapid response to therapy, whereas slower weaning (ie, over a period of months [eg, reducing the total daily dose by 25% every 3 weeks]) is recommended for patients with major problems and/or a long recovery time.[32,38] Should serious side effects be encountered, immediate discontinuation of the drugs can be attempted. Acute discontinuance, however,

---

Box 3
Algorithm for treatment length and weaning schedule

For most psychoactive medications, a treatment period of at least 4 months to 6 months is required, in which the following 4 steps or phases can be distinguished:

1. Treat for the minimum period needed for the drugs to take effect, so that their effect can be assessed. Note that some drugs may have a delayed onset of action, for example:
   • Nonspecific TCAs: minimum 7 days to 10 days
   • More specific TCAs and SSRIs: minimum 3 weeks to 5 weeks

2. Treat until the clinical signs related to the behavior problem have been resolved or at least have been reduced to a low, consistent level
   • Requires an additional period of at least 1 month to 2 months

3. Extend treatment of a similar amount of time it took to attain the level as discussed in (2) to reasonably assure reliability of the assessment.
   • Requires an additional period of at least 1 month to 2 months

4. Taper the drugs off gradually over at least the same amount of time needed for the drugs to take effect (more slowly is also possible, eg, 10–20 days for short-acting psychoactive drugs; 6–8 weeks for longer acting ones).

Note: because reversion of receptor conformation may take 1 month or more, it can take longer before signs are noticed. Although acute weaning off does not necessarily have to result in side effects, full-blown recurrence can occur and is a profound side effect, which is preferably prevented because signs may not resolve after reinitiation of treatment with the same drug and/or the same dose.

Adapted from Overall KL. Pharmacologic treatment in behavioral medicine: the importance of neurochemistry, molecular biology, and mechanistic hypotheses. Vet J 2001;62:18; with permission.

may increase the risk of adverse effects (ie, withdrawal or discontinuation syndrome characterized by rebound anxiety and aggression or reoccurrence of the behavioral problem).[38,56]

Should a favorable response be seen to the medication, weaning of the drug can also be attempted (because ultimately the goal is to not have to use drugs permanently). Prior to attempting to wean a patient off medication, however, it is generally recommended to maintain patients on medication for at least 2 months to 3 months to assure that the effects are long lasting (see **Box 3**). If and when sufficient response to therapy has been ascertained, weaning can be attempted in a similar manner as described previously.

SUMMARY

Although behavior modifying drugs can be useful in the treatment of behavior problems in birds, they are not expected to provide a cure on their own. As a rule, beneficial outcomes can be achieved when using symptom-relieving medication as an adjunct therapy to appropriate behavior modification therapy, environmental adjustments, and adequate treatment of any concurrent medical illnesses. If and when thoughtfully applied, medications are likely to benefit the treatment plan because they can help attenuate an animal's response and increase its receptiveness to the environment. Nevertheless, it is important to remember that each patient is unique and no simple test or specific set of clinical signs exists to determine which drug benefits a patient most. As a result, establishing efficacy of a given treatment regimen in an individual patient largely is based on trial-and-error testing, whereby the initial treatment chosen should always be based on sound rationale regarding the origin of the problem behavior and the prescribed drug's mechanism of action. Moreover, despite the potential added value that hormone therapies and psychoactive drugs can have in the treatment of problem behaviors, it should be considered that drugs can also potentially do harm to a patient when having a negative impact on the treatment plan and/or inducing potential adverse effects. Especially for drugs of which the use has been extrapolated from dogs and cats and on which little information is available in birds, risks of potential side effects are great because a drug's pharmacokinetic and pharmacodynamics profile can vary greatly from that in mammals. As a result, veterinarians are warranted to carefully consider whether medication will benefit the individual patient or not and only consider its use if a beneficial outcome is to be expected.

REFERENCES

1. Gaskins LA, Bergman L. Surveys of avian practitioners and pet owners regarding common behavior problems in psittacine birds. J Avian Med Surg 2011;25:111–8.
2. Symes CT, Perrin MR. Daily flight activity and flocking behaviour patterns of the Greyheaded Parrot *Poicephalus fuscicollis suahelicus* Reichenow 1898 in Northern Province, South Africa. Trop Zool 2003;16:47–62.
3. Bergman L, Reinisch US. Parrot vocalization. In: Luescher AU, editor. Manual of parrot behavior. Ames (IA): Blackwell Publishing; 2006. p. 219–24.
4. Meehan CL, Millam JR, Mench JA. Foraging opportunity and increased physical complexity both prevent and reduce psychogenic feather picking by young Amazon parrots. Appl Anim Behav Sci 2003;80:71–85.
5. Meehan CL, Garner JP, Mench JA. Environmental enrichment and development of cage stereotypy in Orange-winged Amazon parrots (*Amazona amazonica*). Dev Psychobiol 2004;44:209–18.

6. Garner JP, Meehan CL, Famula TR, et al. Genetic, environmental, and neighbor effects on the severity of stereotypies and feather picking in Orange-winged Amazon parrots (*Amazona amazonica*): An epidemiological study. Appl Anim Behav Sci 2006;96:153–68.

7. Mason GJ. Species differences in responses to captivity: stress, welfare and the comparative method. Trends Ecol Evol 2010;25:713–21.

8. Van Zeeland YRA, Spruit BM, Rodenburg TB, et al. Feather damaging behaviour in parrots: A review with consideration of comparative aspects. Appl Anim Behav Sci 2009;121:75–95.

9. Mason G, Clubb R, Latham N, et al. Why and how should we use environmental enrichment to tackle stereotypic behaviour? Appl Anim Behav Sci 2007;102: 163–88.

10. van Zeeland YRA, Friedman SG, Bergman L. Chapter 5-Behavior. In: Speer BL, editor. Current therapy in avian medicine and surgery. St Louis (MO): Elsevier; 2016. p. 177–251.

11. Welle KR, Luescher AU. Aggressive behavior in pet birds. In: Luescher AU, editor. Manual of parrot behavior. Ames (IA): Blackwell Publishing; 2006. p. 211–7.

12. Wilson L, Luescher AU. Parrots and fear. In: Luescher AU, editor. Manual of parrot behavior. Ames (IA): Blackwell Publishing; 2006. p. 225–31.

13. Friedman SG, Haug LI. From parrots to pigs to pythons: universal principles and procedures of learning. Behavior of Exotic Pets. Ames (IA): Wiley-Blackwell; 2010. p. 190–205.

14. Van Sant F. Problem sexual behaviors of companion parrots. In: Luescher AU, editor. Manual of parrot behavior. Ames (IA): Blackwell Publishing; 2006. p. 233–45.

15. Mills DS. Medical paradigms for the study of problem behaviour: a critical review. Appl Anim Behav Sci 2003;81:265–77.

16. Rush AJ, Beck AT, Kovacs M, et al. Comparative efficacy of cognitive therapy and pharmacotherapy in the treatment of depressed outpatients. Cognit Ther Res 1977;1:17–37.

17. DeRubeis RJ, Gelfand LA, Tang TZ, et al. Medications versus cognitive behavior therapy for severely depressed outpatients: mega-analysis of four randomized comparisons. Am J Psychiatry 1999;156:1007–13.

18. Barlow DH, Gorman JM, Shear MK, et al. Cognitive-behavioral therapy, imipramine, or their combination for panic disorder: a randomized controlled trial. JAMA 2000;283:2529–36.

19. Leichsenring F, Leibing E. The effectiveness of psychodynamic therapy and cognitive behavior therapy in the treatment of personality disorders: a meta-analysis. Am J Psychiatry 2003;160:1223–32.

20. Hollon SD, Stewart MO, Strunk D. Enduring effects for cognitive behavior therapy in the treatment of depression and anxiety. Annu Rev Psychol 2006;57: 285–315.

21. Skarphedinsson G, Weidle B, Thomsen PH, et al. Continued cognitive-behavior therapy versus sertraline for children and adolescents with obsessive–compulsive disorder that were non-responders to cognitive-behavior therapy: a randomized controlled trial. Eur child Adolesc Psychiatry 2015;24(5):591–602.

22. Thiébot MH. Some evidence for amnesic-like effects of benzodiazepines in animals. Neurosci Biobehav Rev 1985;9:95–100.

23. Venault P, Chapouthier G, de Carvalho LP, et al. Benzodiazepine impairs and beta-carboline enhances performance in learning and memory tasks. Nature 1986;321:864–6.

24. Nabeshima T, Tohyama K, Ichihara K, et al. Effects of benzodiazepines on passive avoidance response and latent learning in mice: relationship to benzodiazepine receptors and the cholinergic neuronal system. J Pharmacol Exp Ther 1990;255:789–94.

25. Stewart SA. The effects of benzodiazepines on cognition. J Clin Psychiatry 2005;66:9–13.

26. Mason G. Stereotypic behaviour in captive animals: fundamentals and implications for welfare and beyond. In: Mason G, Rushen J, editors. Stereotypic animal behaviour: fundamentals and applications to welfare. 2nd edition. Oxfordshire (United Kingdom): CABI Publishing; 2006. p. 325–56.

27. Garner JP, Meehan CL, Mench JA. Stereotypies in caged parrots, schizophrenia and autism: evidence for a common mechanism. Behav Brain Res 2003;145: 125–34.

28. Shakesby AC, Anwyl R, Rowan MJ. Overcoming the effects of stress on synaptic plasticity in the intact hippocampus: rapid actions of serotonergic and antidepressant agents. J Neurosci 2002;22:3638–44.

29. King JN, Simpson BS, Overall KL, et al. Treatment of separation anxiety in dogs with clomipramine: results from a prospective, randomized, double-blind, placebo-controlled, parallel-group, multicenter clinical trial. Appl Anim Behav Sci 2000;67:255–75.

30. American Psychiatric Association. Diagnostic and statistical manual of mental disorders (DSM-5®). Arlington (VA): American Psychiatric Association; 2013.

31. Schatzberg AF, Debarrista C. Manual of clinical psychopharmacology. Arlington (VA): American Psychiatric Association; 2015.

32. Overall KL. Pharmacological treatment in behavioral medicine: the importance of neurochemistry, molecular biology, and mechanistic hypotheses. Vet J 2001;62:9–23.

33. Friedman SG. A framework for solving behavior problems: functional assessment and intervention planning. J Exot Pet Med 2007;16:6–10.

34. Crowell-Davis SL, Murray T. Veterinary psychopharmacology. Ames (IA): Blackwell Publishing; 2008.

35. Orosz SE. Diagnostic workup of suspected behavioral problems. In: Luescher AU, editor. Manual of parrot behavior. Ames (IA): Blackwell Publishing; 2006. p. 195–210.

36. Welle KR, Wilson L. Clinical evaluation of psittacine behavioral disorders. In: Luescher AU, editor. Manual of parrot behavior. Ames (IA): Blackwell Publishing; 2006. p. 175–93.

37. Mason GJ. Stereotypies—A critical-review. Anim Behav 1991;41:1015–37.

38. Martin KM. Psittacine behavioral pharmacotherapy. In: Luescher AU, editor. Manual of parrot behavior. Ames (IA): Blackwell Publishing; 2006. p. 267–79.

39. Pacher P, Kecskemeti V. Cardiovascular side effects of new antidepressants and antipsychotics: new drugs, old concerns? Curr Pharm Des 2004;10: 2463–75.

40. Kornstein SG, Schatzberg AF, Thase ME, et al. Gender differences in treatment response to sertraline versus imipramine in chronic depression. Am J Psych 2000;157:1445–52.

41. Martényi F, Dossenbach M, Mraz K, et al. Gender differences in the efficacy of fluoxetine and maprotiline in depressed patients: a double-blind trial of antidepressants with serotonergic or norepinephrinergic reuptake inhibition profile. Eur Neuropsychopharmacol 2001;11:227–32.

42. Zandstra SM, Furer JW, Van De Lisdonk EH, et al. Differences in health status between long-term and short-term benzodiazepine users. Br J Gen Pract 2002;52:805–8.
43. Joyce PR, Mulder RT, Luty SE, et al. A differential response to nortriptyline and fluoxetine in melancholic depression: the importance of age and gender. Acta Psychiatr Scand 2003;108:20–3.
44. Khan A, Brodhead AE, Schwartz KA, et al. Sex differences in antidepressant response in recent antidepressant clinical trials. J Clin Psychopharmacol 2005;25:318–24.
45. Van Zeeland YRA, Schoemaker NJ, Haritova A, et al. Pharmacokinetics of paroxetine, a selective serotonin reuptake inhibitor, in Grey parrots (Psittacus erithacus erithacus): influence of pharmaceutical formulation and length of dosing. J Vet Pharmacol Ther 2013;36:51–8.
46. Gruen ME, Sherman BL. Use of trazodone as an adjunctive agent in the treatment of canine anxiety disorders: 56 cases (1995–2007). J Am Vet Med Assoc 2008;233:1902–7.
47. Bauck L. A practitioner's guide to avian medicine. Lakewood (CO): American Animal Hospital Association; 1993.
48. Gaskins LA, Massey JG, Ziccardi MH. Effect of oral diazepam on feeding behavior and activity of Hawaï amakihi (Hemignathus virens). Appl Anim Behav Sci 2008;112:384–94.
49. Carpenter JW. Exotic animal formulary. Ames (IA): Elsevier Health Sciences; 2012.
50. Juarbe-Diaz SJ. Animal behavior case of the month. J Am Vet Med Assoc 2000; 216:1562–4.
51. Welle KR. A review of psychotropic drug therapy. Proceedings of the Annual Conference of the Association of Avian Veterinarians. St. Paul, 1998. p. 121–4.
52. Ramsay EC, Grindlinger H. Use of clomipramine in the treatment of obsessive behavior in psittacine birds. J Assoc Avian Vet 1994;8:9–15.
53. Eugenio CT. Amitriptyline HCl. Clinical study for treatment of feather picking. Proceedings of the Annual Conference of the Association of Avian Veterinarians. Pittsburgh (PA), 2003. p. 133–5.
54. Seibert LM, Crowell-Davis SL, Wilson GH, et al. Placebo-controlled clomipramine trial for the treatment of feather picking disorder in cockatoos. J Am Anim Hosp Assoc 2004;40:261–9.
55. Seibert LM. Pharmacotherapy for behavioral disorders in pet birds. J Exot Pet Med 2007;16:30–7.
56. Visser M, Ragsdale MM, Boothe DM. Pharmacokinetics of amitriptyline HCl and its metabolites in healthy African grey parrots (Psittacus erithacus) and cockatoos (Cacatua species). J Avian Med Surg 2015;29:275–81.
57. Mertens P. Pharmacological treatment of feather picking in pet birds. Proceedings of the First International Meeting of Veterinary Behavioral Medicine, 1997. p. 209–11.
58. Rosenthal K. Psychotrophic agents in pet birds. Proceedings of the North American Veterinary Conference. Florida, 2000. p. 920–1.
59. Wolff MC, Leander JD. Selective serotonin reuptake inhibitors decrease impulsive behavior as measured by an adjusting delay procedure in the pigeon. Neuropsychopharmacology 2002;27:421–9.
60. Kearns K. Paroxetine therapy for feather picking and self-mutilation in the Waldrapp ibis (Geronticus eremita). Proceedings of the Association of Zoo Veterinarians and the American Association of Wildlife Veterinarians, 2004. p. 254–5.

61. Seibert LM. Animal behavior case of the month. J Am Vet Med Assoc 2004;224: 1762–4.

62. Fuchs T, Siegel JJ, Burgdorf J, et al. A selective serotonin reuptake inhibitor reduces REM sleep in the homing pigeon. Physiol Behav 2006;87:575–81.

63. Iglauer F, Rasim R. Treatment of psychogenic leather picking in psittacine birds with a dopamine antagonist. J Small Anim Pract 1993;34:564–6.

64. Lennox A, VanDerHeyden N. Haloperidol for use in treatment of psittacine self-mutilation and feather plucking. Proceedings of the Annual Conference of the Association of Avian Veterinarians. St. Paul, 1993. p. 119–20.

65. Lennox A, VanDerHeyden N. Long-term use of haloperidol in two parrots. Proceedings of the Annual Conference of the Association of Avian Veterinarians. St. Paul, 1993. p. 133–7.

66. Jenkins JR. Feather picking and self-mutilation in psittacine birds. Vet Clin North Am Exot Anim Pract 2001;4:663–7.

67. Turner R. Trexan (naltrexone hydrochloride) use in feather picking in avian species. Proceedings of the Annual Conference of the Association of Avian Veterinarians, 1993. p. 116–8.

68. Crowell-Davis S, Murray T. Benzodiazepines. In: Veterinary psychopharmacology. Ames (IA): Blackwell Publishing; 2006. p. 34–71.

69. Mans C, Guzman DSM, Lahner LL, et al. Sedation and physiologic response to manual restraint after intranasal administration of midazolam in Hispaniolan Amazon parrots (Amazona ventralis). J Avian Med Surg 2012;26:130–9.

70. File SE. The history of benzodiazepine dependence: a review of animal studies. Neurosci Biobehav Rev 1990;14:135–46.

71. Petursson H. The benzodiazepine withdrawal syndrome. Addiction 1994;89: 1455–9.

72. Ninan PT, Cole JO, Yonkers KA. Nonbenzodiazepine anxiolytics. In: Schatzberg AF, Nemeroff CB, editors. The American psychiatric press textbook of psychopharmacology. 2nd edition. Washington, DC: American Psychiatric Press; 1998. p. 287–300.

73. Crowell-Davis S, Murray T. Azapirones. In: Veterinary psychopharmacology. Ames (IA): Blackwell Publishing; 2006. p. 111–8.

74. Eison AS, Temple DL. Buspirone: review of its pharmacology and current perspectives on its mechanism of action. Am J Med 1986;80:1–9.

75. Pohl R, Balon R, Yeragani VK, et al. Serotonergic anxiolytics in the treatment of panic disorder: a controlled study with buspirone. Psychopathology 1989; 22(Suppl 1):60–7.

76. Ratey J, Sovner R, Parks A, et al. Buspirone treatment of aggression and anxiety in mentally retarded patients: a multiple-baseline, placebo lead-in study. J Clin Psychiatry 1991;52:159–62.

77. Kehne JH, Cassella JV, Davis M. Anxiolytic effects of buspirone and gepirone in the fear-potentiated startle paradigm. Psychopharmacology (Berl) 1988;94:8–13.

78. Lucki I, Rickels K, Giesecke MA, et al. Differential effects of the anxiolytic drugs, diazepam and buspirone, on memory function. Br J Clin Pharmacol 1987;23: 207–11.

79. Crowell-Davis S, Murray T. Tricyclic antidepressants. In: Veterinary psychopharmacology. Ames (IA): Blackwell Publishing; 2006. p. 179–206.

80. Hewson CJ, Luescher UA, Parent JM, et al. Efficacy of clomipramine in the treatment of canine compulsive disorder. J Am Vet Med Assoc 1998;213:1760–6.

81. Overall KL, Dunham AE. Clinical features and outcome in dogs and cats with obsessive-compulsive disorder: 126 cases (1989–2000). J Am Vet Med Assoc 2002;221:1445–52.

82. Johnson C. Chronic feather picking: a different approach to treatment. Proceedings of the Annual Conference of the Association of Avian Veterinarians, 1987. p. 125–42.

83. Starkey SR, Morrisey JK, Hickam HD, et al. Extrapyramidal side effects in a Blue and gold macaw (*Ara ararauna*) treated with haloperidol and clomipramine. J Avian Med Surg 2008;22:234–9.

84. Crowell-Davis S, Murray T. Selective serotonin reuptake inhibitors. In: Veterinary psychopharmacology. Ames (IA): Blackwell Publishing; 2006. p. 80–110.

85. Hyttel J. Pharmacological characterization of selective serotonin reuptake inhibitors (SSRIs). Int Clin Psychopharmacol 1994;9:19–26.

86. Anderson IM. Selective serotonin reuptake inhibitors versus tricyclic antidepressants: a meta-analysis of efficacy and tolerability. J Affect Disord 2000;58: 19–36.

87. Brambilla P, Cipriani A, Hotopf M, et al. Side-effect profile of fluoxetine in comparison with other SSRIs, tricyclic and newer antidepressants: a meta-analysis of clinical trial data. Pharmacopsychiatry 2005;38:69–77.

88. Crowell-Davis S, Murray T. Antipsychotics. In: Veterinary psychopharmacology. Ames (IA): Blackwell Publishing; 2006. p. 148–65.

89. Luescher A. Compulsive behavior: recognition and treatment. Proceedings of the Annual Conference of the American Association of Zoo Veterinarians, 1998. p. 398–402.

90. Crowell-Davis S, Murray T. Opioids and opioid antagonists. In: Veterinary psychopharmacology. Ames (IA): Blackwell Publishing; 2006. p. 212–23.

91. Brown S, Crowell-Davis S, Malcolm T, et al. Naloxone-responsive compulsive tail chasing in a dog. J Am Vet Med Assoc 1987;190:884–6.

92. Dodman NH, Shuster L, White SD, et al. Use of narcotic antagonists to modify stereotypic self-licking, self-chewing, and scratching behavior in dogs. J Am Vet Med Assoc 1988;193:815–9.

93. White SD. Naltrexone for treatment of acral lick dermatitis in dogs. J Am Vet Med Assoc 1990;196:1073–6.

94. Kenny DE. Use of naltrexone for treatment of psychogenically induced dermatoses in five zoo animals. J Am Vet Med Assoc 1994;205:1021–3.

95. Dodman NH, Shuster D. Psychopharmacology of animal behavior disorders. Malden (MA): Blackwell Science; 1998.

96. Forbes NA. The use of GnRH implants in the treatment of sexual derived behavioural abnormalities in birds. Proceedings of the Bi-annual Conference of the European Association of Avian Veterinarians and the European College of Zoological Medicine, 2009. p. 119–22.

97. Pollock CG, Orosz SE. Avian reproductive anatomy, physiology and endocrinology. Vet Clin North Am Exot Anim Pract 2002;5:441–74.

98. Ottinger MA, Wu J, Pelican K. Neuroendocrine regulation of reproduction in birds and clinical applications of GnRH analogues in birds and mammals. Sem Avian Exot Pet Med 2002;11(2):71–9.

99. Mans C, Pilny A. Use of GnRH-agonists for medical management of reproductive disorders in birds. Vet Clin North Am Exot Anim Pract 2014;17:23–33.

100. Zantop D. Using leuprolide acetate to manage common avian reproductive problems. Exotic DVM 2000;2:70.

101. Powers LV. Clinical use of melatonin in birds. Proceedings of the Exoticscon Conference in 2015 - Joint conference of the Association of Avian Veterinarians, Association of Exotic Mammal Veterinarians and Association of Reptile and Amphibian Veterinarians, 2016. p. 297–302.

102. McGuire NL, Kangas K, Bentley GE. Effects of melatonin on peripheral reproductive function: Regulation of testicular GnIH and testosterone. Endocrinology 2011;152:3461–70.

103. Sladky KK, Krugner-Higby L, Meek-Walker E, et al. Serum concentrations and analgesic effects of liposome-encapsulated and standard butorphanol tartrate in parrots. American journal of veterinary research 2006;67(5):775–81.

104. Hawkins MG, Paul-Murphy J, Guzman DSM. Recognition, assessment, and management of pain in birds. In: Speer BL, editor. Current therapy in avian medicine and surgery. St Louis (MO): Elsevier; 2016. p. 616–30.

105. Doneley B. The use of gabapentin to treat presumed neuralgia in a little corella (*Cacatua sanguinea*). Proceedings of the Australasian Association of Avian Veterinarians, 2007. p. 169–72.

106. Siperstein LJ. Use of Neurontin (gabapentin) to treat leg twitching/foot mutilation in a Senegal parrot. Proceedings of the Annual Conference of the Association of Avian Veterinarians, 2007. p. 81–2.

107. Shaver SL, Robinson NG, Wright BD, et al. A multimodal approach to management of suspected neuropathic pain in a prairie falcon (*Falco mexicanus*). J Avian Med Surg 2009;23:209–13.

108. Taylor CP. Mechanisms of analgesia by gabapentin and pregabalin—calcium channel α2-δ [Cavα2-δ] ligands. Pain 2009;142:13–6.

109. Baine K, Jones MP, Cox S, et al. Pharmacokinetics of compounded intravenous and oral gabapentin in Hispaniolan Amazon parrots (*Amazona ventralis*). J Avian Med Surg 2015;29:165–73.

110. Yaw TJ, Zaffarano BA, Gall A, et al. Pharmacokinetic properties of a single administration of oral gabapentin in the great horned owl (*Bubo virginianus*). J Zoo Wildl Med 2015;463:547–52.

111. McLean MJ, Morrell MJ, Willmore LJ, et al. Safety and tolerability of gabapentin as adjunctive therapy in a large, multicenter study. Epilepsia 1999;40:965–72.

112. Colombini S, Foil CS, Hosgood G, et al. Intradermal skin testing in Hispaniolan parrots (*Amazona ventralis*). Vet Dermatol 2000;11:271–6.

113. Rosenthal KL, Morris DO, Mauldin EA, et al. Cytologic, histologic, and microbiologic characterization of the feather pulp and follicles of feather-picking psittacine birds: a preliminary study. J Avian Med Surg 2004;18:137–43.

114. Garner MM, Clubb SL, Mitchell MA, et al. Feather-picking psittacines: histopathology and species trends. Vet Pathol 2008;45:401–8.

115. Scott D, Miller W. Antihistamines in the management of allergic pruritus in dogs and cats. J Small Anim Pract 1999;40:359–64.

116. Krinsley M. Use of dermcaps liquid and hydroxyzine HCl for the treatment of feather picking. J Assoc Avian Vet 1993;7:221.

117. Westerhof I, Pellicaan CH. Effects of different application routes of glucocorticoids on the pituitary-adrenocortical axis in pigeons (*Columba livia domestica*). J Avian Med Surg 1995;9:175–81.

118. Delk K. Clinical management of seizures in avian patients. J Exot Pet Med 2012; 21:132–9.

119. Sadock BJ, Sadock VA. Kaplan and Sadock's pocket handbook of clinical psychiatry. Philadelphia: Lippincott Williams & Wilkins; 2010.

120. Aranow A, Hudson JI, Pope HG Jr, et al. Elevated antidepressant plasma levels after addition of fluoxetine. Am J Psychiatry 1989;146:911–3.
121. Powers LV, Papich MG. Pharmacokinetics of orally administered phenobarbital in African grey parrots (*Psittacus erithacus erithacus*). J Vet Pharmacol Ther 2011;34:615–7.
122. Beaufrère H, Nevarez J, Gaschen L, et al. Diagnosis of presumed acute ischemic stroke and associated seizure management in a Congo African grey parrot. J Am Vet Med Assoc 2011;239:122–8.
123. Schnellbacher R, Beaufrere H, Vet DM, et al. Pharmacokinetics of levetiracetam in healthy Hispaniolan Amazon parrots (*Amazona ventralis*) after oral administration of a single dose. J Avian Med Surg 2014;28:193–200.
124. Visser M, Boothe DM. Population pharmacokinetics of levetiracetam and zonisamide in the African grey parrot (*Psittacus erithacus*). Proceedings of the Exoticscon Conference, 2015. p. 7–10.

Functional and Anatomic Correlates of Neural Aging in Birds

Mary Ann Ottinger, BS, MS, PhD

KEYWORDS

- Neural aging • Neuroendocrine system aging • Long- and short-lived birds • Aging

KEY POINTS

- Short-lived birds experience reproductive aging, with declining endocrine and neuroendocrine function and behavioral alterations.
- Long-lived birds show negligible reproductive decline; however, there is evidence of behavioral and cognitive changes in individuals.
- Conserved mechanisms underlie age-related changes in the avian brain similar to those observed in mammals suggesting conserved mechanisms for overall aging processes.

INTRODUCTION

Avian species (class Aves) are among the most ubiquitous vertebrates, spanning the globe in a variety of habitats and adaptations. In addition to great variation in lifetime reproductive, physiologic, and adaptive strategies, birds have a number of unique characteristics that allow them to migrate great distances and survive under highly variable and sometimes extreme conditions.[1] More impressive, avian species have a higher metabolism, body temperature, and unique bone and air sac structure to enhance flight capability. Moreover, it would be predicted that the higher body temperature and metabolic rate would result in a shorter lifespan. Many birds, including several species of hummingbirds, parrots, and seabirds, exhibit remarkably long lifespans.[2–8] Although there is evidence that long-lived birds reduced oxidative damage compared with short-lived birds, age-related diseases also occur including cardiovascular disease, cancer, osteoarthritis, and endocrine system decline. This review coalesces the available literature on the aging of neural systems in birds, with a focus on functional impacts as the aging process progresses.

The author has nothing to disclose; research supported by NRI #92-37203 and NSF #9817024 to M.A. Ottinger.
Department of Biology and Biochemistry, University of Houston, 4302 University Drive, Room 316, Houston, TX 77204, USA
E-mail address: maotting@central.uh.edu

AN OVERVIEW OF AGING IN BIRDS

There is a very large literature on domestic birds, including many studies that have provided critical information to the poultry industry for the optimization of productivity, breeding and genetics, and disease prevention and management. These studies have also greatly contributed to the overall understanding of the fundamental biology of avian species. Studies in domestic species have concentrated on declining productivity, especially in egg production and fertility as the flock ages.[9-13] Initial studies showed that the characteristics of this age-related decrease in egg production included decreasing egg production accompanied by thinning eggshell, with little discernable change in circulating steroids.[14] Further, the timing in this age-related decline in aging varies with strain of domestic chick in that the Leghorn hens continued high egg production while the heavier Rhode Island Red line showed decreasing egg production with longer interoviposition intervals.[10] Coincident with the declining egg production, other indicators of age-related decline begin to emerge including alterations in neuroendocrine response, shell quality decline, and increasing evidence of metabolic system changes.[9,11-13] Osteoporosis often presents severe problems for aging poultry, especially in egg-laying strains that may produce 300 or more eggs per year. The bones of female birds generally serve as a repository for calcium and other minerals needed for egg production. Female quail develop increasingly fragile bones as they age and have served as an excellent model for poultry layers in understanding the effects of hormones and dietary treatments on.[15] There is evidence that the availability of perches alleviates as well as improves bone and muscle health in egg laying birds.[16] This finding is similar to a large literature in humans and other mammals that reinforce the beneficial effects of exercise, especially weight-bearing exercise on bone health and muscle functionality. Finally, birds with high egg production have a high incidence of ovarian cancers, likely associated with the extensive rupture repair processes with daily ovulations. As such, poultry have an excellent model understanding some of the basic biology of osteoporosis and ovarian cancer.

Short-lived male birds also show evidence of aging, particularly in endocrine and behavioral components of reproduction.[17,18] This includes decreased sperm production and increased sperm abnormalities over time.[11,19] Interestingly, male brain retains plasticity during aging as demonstrated by responsiveness to exogenous testosterone replacement in reproductively senescent males by recovery of reproductive function, including function of specific neuropeptide pathways in the hypothalamus regulating sexual behavior and gonadotropin-releasing hormone. This response, in turn, allows for the investigation of the roles of these molecules in the aging brain–gonadal system.

A number of studies have also focused on short- and long-lived avian species to understand mechanisms underlying the process of aging and also to investigated biomarkers as indices of aging status. The comparison of putative biomarkers has provided valuable information for ascertaining if conserved mechanisms in aging processes span across vertebrate and even invertebrate species. Some of these mechanisms include altered immune system function and other markers of the aging process that seem to occur in tandem with reproductive endocrine decline.[6,8] Further, the link between environmental stressors and healthy aging is clearly critical, affecting both health and longevity.[20] Cellular markers, specifically telomeres and the influence of oxidative damage, have received a great deal of attention, both as bioindicators and contributors to age-related demise in physiologic systems. Species comparisons have shown that avian telomeric DNA sequences are longer than in mammals; however, average telomere length and maximum life span did not seem to be related.[21] Aydinonat and colleagues[22] demonstrated that telomere length decreased with age and socially isolated African Gray parrots had even shorter telomeres than communally housed birds of the same age. Haussmann and Heidinger[23] present evidence that stressors may play a critical role, both in adults and offspring in terms of aging and telomere dynamics. Along these lines, the adverse impact of oxidative damage has received attention as a potential trigger for age-related cellular breakdown. Moreover, short-lived birds show less resistance to damage from oxidative damage compared with long-lived birds.[24–27] However, contradictory evidence showing no difference in oxidative damage and associated cellular metabolic processes have been reported by Montgomery and colleagues.[28–30] Interestingly, there is evidence for differential cellular responses to oxidative stress accompanying atherosclerosis: quail microvascular endothelial cells show greater resilience by production of heme oxygenase as protection against oxidized lipids.[31] Taken together, these processes are complex and there is intriguing evidence for a differential and potentially advantageous mechanisms, especially in long-lived birds. Additional studies to clarify processes associated with aging versus those that may not related to longevity. As such and not unexpectedly, the process of aging is not only complex yet variable on an individual basis making it difficult to discern clear initiators or even the involved pathways leading to senescence.

EVIDENCE OF NEURAL AND COGNITIVE AGING IN SHORT- AND LONG-LIVED BIRDS

Birds have relatively large brains compared with other taxa, with a vast array of variation across the species.[32] Data from field studies provide insight into age-related adaptations and behavioral variations, but do not directly address learning or cognition. Common terns show age-dependent breeding patterns with extended reproductive competency in breeding pairs continuing to produce successful fledglings to more than 20 years of age.[5,7,33] Further, longer lived individuals began breeding earlier and maintained reproduction longer.[34] In the wandering albatross, females had continued breeding success longer than males.[35] At a theoretic level, Ricklefs[36] suggested linage between rates of maturation and aging, with slowly maturing species having greater longevity. Salient to this question, Finch and colleagues[37] have coalesced data across a number of vertebrate species to capture overarching tenants impacting lifetime patterns and mechanisms in aging. Some key elements, such as inflammation, stress response, physiologic resilience, and oxidative damage continue to emerge as linked to aging and lifespan.[38] Examination of these elements in tandem with understanding slowly aging organisms will further elucidate initiators and mechanisms operating in the progression of age-related decline.[39] Birds in captivity as pets or in zoologic parks provide a permissive environment for individuals to achieve maximal lifespan. As these birds age, they experience physiologic and pathologic processes that impact their overall health, allowing observation of aging processes.[40] Specific studies of neural and cognitive aging have not received a great deal of attention in birds, especially from the standpoint of clinical studies of captive species; an overview of these studies follows.

Auditory and Visual System Aging

Aging of auditory and visual systems reflects both sensory and neural integration and these systems have been studied in detail. Interestingly, aging quail experience a loss of ganglion cell number during aging.[41] However, quail also retain an ability to regenerate hair cells, even after damage has been inflicted throughout the life span.[42,43] Visual system aging is a key component in the decline of productivity, because photoperiodic sensing relies on both on retinal projections to the midbrain synergizing with melatonin produced by the pineal gland. Diminished response to photoperiodic cues leads to photorefractoriness and diminished reproduction, which becomes a critical factor in productivity of poultry breeding flocks. Beyond production implications, visual system aging has been observed in pigeons with age-related declining visual threshold perception, which contributes with diminished discrimination tasks.[44] This, in combination with diminished visual acuity and loss of photoreceptors in the ganglion cell layer of the retina, contribute to the aging of the visual system.[45] Finally, an in-depth study of pigeons up to 20 years of age revealed a bimodal decline in visual acuity with an initial loss by 8 years of age followed by a gradual decline, possibly owing to choroidal vascular decline.[46] Taken together, it is clear that both auditory and visual systems show age-related declines that can impact performance in learning and memory.

Cognitive Function and Aging

There is a fascinating array of cognitive behaviors across avian species, with unique problem solving and tool use in some field species. The New Caledonian crow has been shown to be an excellent tool user.[47,48] Given the evidence that birds learn language and exhibit other behaviors involving remembering location of a cache or problem solving suggests that birds might provide excellent models for understanding the fundamentals of cognitive function.[49,50] An overview of episodic-like memory across avian species reveals a range of adaptive approaches in cognition used by birds.[51] The western scrub-jay shows an ability to problem solve tasks involving choice to obtain a reward.[52] Long-term study of individuals using problem solving will provide insights into the ability for birds to continue using adaptive cognitive processes throughout their lifespan and if these capabilities diminish with aging.

Domesticated birds provide in-depth insights into cognitive capabilities, especially through laboratory studies. It has been argued that social behavior and social interactions in domestic poultry are also indicative of cognitive function.[53] Stress impacted performance of aged Japanese quail on spatial memory tasks, suggesting that both episodic and chronic stressors have adverse effects on cognitive performance.[54] Pigeons have served as excellent avian models for learning and memory studies; age-related impairment has been described for spatial memory performance in which older pigeons were more stereotypic in their responses and required more time to complete tasks to criterion.[55] In pigeons, as in other birds, the hippocampus is a critical area in learning and memory. In homing pigeons, neurogenesis was greatest in young birds and declined with advancing age.[56] In separate studies, the key role of the hippocampus formation in spatial perception was also deemed critical for navigation and spatial perception.[57] Long-lived parrots show an uncanny ability to learn and articulate words in the proper intonation and context. These long-lived birds may show behavioral change over time in an individual; however, few clinically documented studies exist.

SUMMARY

Avian species demonstrate a vast array of lifetime adaptations to meet the demands of environmental challenges. Some birds have extended lifespan by living in cooperative societal social structures.[58] Further, it has been shown that environmental conditions in early life may impact long-term survival.[59] Neurotransmitter and neuroendocrine systems are a clear and key component of age-related decline in endocrine function and behavioral responses.[7,11,60,61] As more data are gathered, it will be important to discern between the observed differences in lifetime patterns resulting from of deteriorating physiologic processes or if there are initiating events of dysregulation of rhythmic patterns ultimately disrupting the myriad of interlinked functional processes. As we learn more, it will then be possible to distinguish predicted age-related changes as apposed to disease conditions. This will be critical to formulate appropriate treatments and interventions as well as proactively construct regimens to clinically recognize and potential forestall deleterious physiologic changes.

REFERENCES

1. Gill FB. Ornithology. 2nd edition. New York: W.H. Freeman and Co; 1995.
2. Holmes DJ, Ottinger MA. Domestic and wild bird models for the study of aging. In: Michael Conn P, editor. Handbook of models for human aging. Amsterdam: Elsevier; 2006. p. 351–66.
3. Holmes DJ, Ottinger MA. Biology of aging in Avian species. Special Issue of the American Aging Association Journal 2003;27:1–5.
4. Holmes DJ, Thomson SL, Wu J, et al. Reproductive aging in female birds. Exp Gerontol 2003;38(7):751–6.
5. Nisbet ICT, Finch CE, Thompson N, et al. Endocrine patterns during aging in the common tern (Sterna hirundo). Gen Comp Endocrinol 1999;114:279–86.
6. Ottinger MA, Lavoie E. Neuroendocrine and immune characteristics of aging in avian species. Cytogenet Genome Res 2007;117(1–4):352–7.
7. Ottinger MA, Nisbet ICT, Finch CE. Aging and reproduction: comparative endocrinology of the common tern and Japanese quail. Am Zoologist 1995;35: 299–306.
8. Ottinger MA, Ricklefs RE, Finch CE. Proceedings of the 2nd Symposium on organisms with slow aging (SOSA-2). Exp Gerontol 2003;38(7):1–2.
9. Ciccone NA, Sharp PJ, Wilson PW, et al. Changes in reproductive neuroendocrine mRNAs with decreasing ovarian function in ageing hens. Gen Comp Endocrinol 2005;144(1):20–7.
10. Lillpers K, Wilhelmson M. Age-dependent changes in oviposition pattern and egg production traits in the domestic hen. Poult Sci 1993;72(11):2005–11.
11. Ottinger MA. Altered neuroendocrine mechanisms during reproductive aging. Poult Sci Rev 1992;4:235–48.
12. Robinson FE, Hardin RT, Robblee AR. Reproductive senescence in domestic fowl; effects on egg production, sequence length and inter-sequence pause length. Br Poult Sci 1990;31(4):871–9.
13. Sharp PJ, Dunn IC, Cerolini S. Neuroendocrine control of reduced persistence of egg-laying in domestic hens: evidence for the development of photorefractoriness. J Reprod Fertil 1992;94(1):221–35.
14. Joyner CJ, Peddie MJ, Taylor TG. The effect of age on egg production in the domestic hen. Gen Comp Endocrinol 1987;65(3):331–6.
15. Kaetzel DM Jr, Soares JH Jr. Effect of dietary calcium stress on plasma vitamin D3 metabolites in the egg-laying Japanese quail. Poult Sci 1985;64(4):1121–7.
16. Hester PY, Enneking SA, Haley BK, et al. The effect of perch availability during pullet rearing and egg laying on musculoskeletal health of caged White Leghorn hens. Poult Sci 2013;92(8):1972–80.
17. Ottinger MA. Neuroendocrine and behavioral determinants of reproductive aging. CRC Reviews Poultry Biology 1991;3:131–42.
18. Ottinger MA. Quail and other short-lived birds. Experimental Gerontology 2001; 36(4–6):859–68.
19. Ottinger MA. Aging in the Avian brain: neuroendocrine considerations. Semin Avian Exot Pet Med 1996;5(3):172–7.

20. Nelson BF, Daunt F, Monaghan P, et al. Protracted treatment with corticosterone reduces breeding success in a long-lived bird. Gen Comp Endocrinol 2015;210: 38045.

21. Delany ME, Krupkin AB, Miller MM. Organization of telomere sequences in birds: evidence for arrays of extreme length and for in vivo shortening. Cytogenet Cell Genet 2000;90:139–45.

22. Aydinonat D, Penn DJ, Smith S, et al. Social isolation shortens telomeres in African Grey parrots (Psittacus erithacus erithacus). PLoS One 2014;9(4):e93839.

23. Haussmann MF, Heidinger BJ. Telomere dynamics may link stress exposure and ageing across generations. Biol Lett 2015;11(11) [pii:20150396].

24. Herrero A, Barja G. 8-oxo-deoxyguanosine levels in heart and brain mitochondrial and nuclear DNA of two mammals and three birds in relation to their different rates of aging. Aging (Milano) 1999;11(5):294–300.

25. Ogburn CE, Austad SN, Holmes DJ, et al. Cultured renal epithelial cells from birds and mice: enhanced resistance of avian cells to oxidative stress and DNA damage. J Gerontol A Biol Sci Med Sci 1998;53A:B287–92.

26. Ogburn CE, Martin GM, Ottinger MA, et al. Exceptional cellular resistance to oxidative damage in long-lived birds requires active gene expression. J Gerontol Biol Sci 2001;11:B468–74.

27. Pamplona R, Portero-Otín M, Riba D, et al. Heart fatty acid unsaturation and lipid peroxidation, and aging rate, are lower in the canary and the parakeet than in the mouse. Aging (Milano) 1999;11:44–9.

28. Montgomery MK, Buttemer WA, Hulbert AJ. Does the oxidative stress theory of aging explain longevity differences in birds? II. Antioxidant systems and oxidative damage. Exp Gerontol 2012;47(3):211–22.

29. Montgomery MK, Hulbert AJ, Buttemer WA. Does the oxidative theory of aging explain longevity differences in birds? I. Mitochondrial ROS production. Exp Gerontol 2012;47(3):203–10.

30. Montgomery MK, Hulbert AJ, Buttemer WA. Metabolic rate and membrane fatty acid composition in birds: a comparison between long-living parrots and short-living fowl. J Comp Physiol B 2012;182(1):127–37.

31. Hoekstra KA, Velleman SG. Brain microvascular and intracranial artery resistance to atherosclerosis is associated with heme oxygenase and ferritin in Japanese quail. Mol Cell Biochem 2008;307(1–2):1–12.

32. Isler K, Van Schaik CP. Why are there so few smart mammals (but so many smart birds)? Biol Lett 2009;5(1):125–9.

33. Breton AR, Nisbet ICT, Mostello CS, et al. Age-dependent breeding dispersal and adult survival within a metapopulation of Common Terns Sterna hirundo. IBIS 2014;156:534–47.

34. Zhang H, Vedder O, Becker PH, et al. Age-dependent trait variation: the relative contribution of within-individual change, selective appearance and disappearance in a long-lived seabird. J Anim Ecol 2015;84(3):797–807.

35. Pardo D, Barbraud C, Weimerskirch H. Females better face senescence in the wandering albatross. Oecologia 2013;173(4):1283–94.

36. Ricklefs RE. Life-history connections to rates of aging in terrestrial vertebrates. Proc Natl Acad Sci U S A 2010;107(22):10314–9.

37. Finch CE, Crimmins EM. Constant molecular aging rates vs. the exponential acceleration of mortality. Proc Natl Acad Sci U S A 2016;113(5):1121–3.

38. Finch CE, Morgan TE, Longo VD, et al. Cell resilience in species life spans: a link to inflammation? Aging Cell 2010;9(4):519–26. Fi.

39. Finch CE. Update on slow aging and negligible senescence—a mini-review. Gerontology 2009;55(3):307–13.
40. Reavill DR, Dorrestein GM. Pathology of aging psittacines. Vet Clin North Am Exot Anim Pract 2010;13(1):135–50.
41. Ryals BM, Westbrook EW. Ganglion cell and hair cell loss in Coturnix quail associated with aging. Hear Res 1988;36(1):1–8.
42. Ryals BM, Westbrook EW. Hair cell regeneration in senescent quail. Hear Res 1990;50(1–2):87–96.
43. Ryals BM, Westbrook EW. TEM analysis of neural terminals on autoradiographically identified regenerated hair cells. Hear Res 1994;72(1–2):81–8.
44. Kurkjian ML, Hodos W. Age-dependent intensity-difference thresholds in pigeons. Vision Res 1992;32(7):1249–52.
45. Hodos W, Miller RF, Fite KV. Age-dependent changes in visual acuity and retinal morphology in pigeons. Vision Res 1991;31(4):669–77.
46. Fitzgerald ME, Tolley E, Frase S, et al. Functional and morphological assessment of age-related changes in the choroid and outer retina in pigeons. Vis Neurosci 2001;18(2):299–317.
47. Rutz C, Klump BC, Komarczyk L, et al. Discovery of species-wide tool use in the Hawaiian crow. Nature 2016;537(7620):403–7.
48. Uomini N, Hunt G. A new tool-using bird to crow about. Learn Behav 2017. [Epub ahead of print].
49. Clayton NS, Emery NJ. Avian models for human cognitive neuroscience: a proposal. Neuron 2015;86(6):1330–42.
50. Watanabe A, Clayton NS. Hint-seeking behavior of western scrub-jays in a meta-cognition task. Anim Cogn 2016;19(1):53–64.
51. Salwiczek LH, Watanabe A, Clayton NS. Ten years of research into avian models of episodic-like memory and its implications for developmental and comparative cognition. Behav Brain Res 2010;215(2):221–34.
52. Hofmann MM, Cheke LG, Clayton NS. Western scrub-jays (*Aphelocoma californica*) solve multiple-string problems by the spatial relation of string and reward. Anim Cogn 2016;19(6):1103–14.
53. Marino L. Thinking chickens: a review of cognition, emotion, and behavior in the domestic chicken. Anim Cogn 2017;20(2):127–47.
54. Suhr CL, Schmidt JB, Treese ST, et al. Short-term spatial memory responses in aged Japanese quail selected for divergent adrenocortical stress responsiveness. Pout Sci 2010;89(4):633–42.
55. Coppola VJ, Hough G, Bingman VP. Age-related spatial deficits in homing pigeons (*Columba livia*). Behav Neurosci 2014;128(6):666–75.
56. Meskenaite V, Krackow S, Lipp HP. Age-dependent neurogenesis and neuron numbers within the olfactory bulb and hippocampus of homing pigeons. Front Behav Neurosci 2016;10:126.
57. Herold C, Coppola VJ, Bingman VP. The maturation of research into the avian hippocampal formation: recent discoveries from one of nature's foremost navigators. Hippocampus 2015;25(11):1193–211.
58. Downing PA, Cornawallis CK, Griffin AS. Sex, long life and the evolutionary transition to cooperative breeding in birds. Proc Biol Sci 2015;282(1816):20151663.
59. Balbontin J, Moller AP. Environmental conditions during early life accelerate the rate of senescence in a short-lived passerine bird. Ecology 2015;96(4):948–59.

60. Avital-Cohen N, Heiblum R, Rosenstrauch A, et al. Role of the serotonergic axis in the reproductive failure associated with aging broiler breeder roosters. Domest Anim Endocrinol 2015;53:42–51.

61. Ottinger MA, Corbitt C, Hoffman R, et al. Reproductive aging in Japanese quail, Coturnix japonica is associated with changes in central opioid receptors. Brain Res 2006;1126(1):167–75.

Gut Brain Axis and Its Microbiota Regulation in Mammals and Birds

Jan S. Suchodolski, MedVet, DrMedVet, PhD, DACVM

KEYWORDS

• Microbiota • Microbiome • Bacteria • Gut-brain-axis • Serotonin

KEY POINTS

- The intestine harbors a highly complex microbial ecosystem consisting of bacteria, fungi, viruses, and parasites.
- Bacterial culture and fecal cytology does not allow proper assessment of intestinal bacteria, and molecular-based methods are now standard in the assessment of bacterial microbiota.
- The intestinal microbiota is a highly active immunologic and metabolomic system that is crucial to host health.
- Various microbiota-derived metabolites contribute to neuroendocrine pathways that provide signaling to the brain via the gut-brain axis.

INTESTINAL MICROBIOTA AND ITS FUNCTION

The intestinal microbiota is defined as the collection of all living microbes (bacteria, fungi, protozoa, and viruses) residing in the gastrointestinal (GI) tract. Until a decade ago, bacterial culture was the most commonly used technique to describe bacteria within the mammalian and avian GI tract. The recent advance of molecular tools, especially next-generation sequencing technologies that allow to inexpensively amplify, sequence, and thereby identify which bacterial taxa are present in a sample, has revolutionized understanding and revealed that the GI microbiota of mammals and birds is much more species-rich than previously thought.[1] In mammals, it is estimated that 100 trillion bacterial cells populate the GI tract and the total sum of bacteria is approximately 10 times more than the number of host cells. The collective genome of all these microbes (referred to as microbiome) exists in close relationship with the host and, through its immunologic and metabolic function, this highly complex microbial-host ecosystem has a crucial impact on host health, including the nervous system.

Disclosure Statement: The author has nothing to disclose.
Small Animal Medicine, Gastrointestinal Laboratory, Department of Small Animal Clinical Sciences, Texas A&M University, 4474 TAMU, College Station, TX 77843-4474, USA
E-mail address: Jsuchodolski@cvm.tamu.edu

Vet Clin Exot Anim 21 (2018) 159–167
http://dx.doi.org/10.1016/j.cvex.2017.08.007
1094-9194/18/© 2017 Elsevier Inc. All rights reserved.

vetexotic.theclinics.com

Resident bacteria provide many beneficial mechanisms, such as fending off transient enteropathogens, aiding in nutrition and harvesting energy from diet, providing metabolites that feed enterocytes, and stimulating the host immune system. Although most data about the functions of the intestinal microbiota are derived from studies in mammals and fewer data are available in avian species, it is likely that many microbiota–host interactions are evolutionary and conserved across various animal species. For example, in mammals, complex fibers obtained through the diet (eg, starch, cellulose, pectin) are fermented by intestinal bacteria. The end products of this bacterial fermentation are short-chain fatty acids (SCFA). These are partially absorbed and serve as an energy source for the host (eg, propionate, acetate), regulate intestinal motility, and are also used as important growth factors for the intestinal epithelial cells. SCFA are also important stimuli for maintaining intestinal barrier function, thereby minimizing bacterial translocation.[2,3] SCFA are also immunomodulatory by activing regulatory T cells in the intestine.[4] Although SCFA are the most studied bacterially derived metabolites, novel metabolomics approaches have revealed various other metabolites that are produced by intestinal microbiota, such as indole, a byproduct of tryptophan degradation, which is anti-inflammatory and enhances intestinal barrier function.[5] Of importance is that bacterial metabolism and immunologic stimulation in the intestine have consequences that reach far beyond the GI tract. It is now well-recognized that a gut-brain connection exists that is modulated by gut microbes. Modulation of gut microbiota is an exciting emerging area of research with the potential for better understanding of pathophysiology and treatment of various intestinal and metabolic, as well as neurologic diseases.

ASSESSMENT OF INTESTINAL MICROBIOTA

Until a decade ago, most information about the composition of the intestinal microbiota was obtained using traditional culturing techniques. Bacterial culture is a useful tool for determination of an active infection of known pathogens (eg, *Salmonella*, *Campylobacter*) and antibiotic susceptibility testing in clinical specimens. Individual isolates and their virulence factors can be typed for epidemiologic surveys of specific strains. It is now well-recognized that there are several limitations associated with bacterial culture of intestinal samples. Bacterial culture widely underestimates the total bacterial numbers in the intestines. Most gut bacteria cannot be isolated on routinely used laboratory media because not enough information is available about their optimal growth requirements. Most microbes in the gut are strict facultative anaerobes, hindering their successful isolation in vitro. It is estimated that less than 10% of intestinal bacteria can be cultured on routine media and only a small fraction can be correctly classified using classic morphologic and biochemical criteria. Therefore, clinical examination of intestinal samples by culture is currently biased toward the minor cultivable portion of the gut microbiota.

Because of these limitations, the use of molecular tools is now standard. The principle is that DNA is extracted from intestinal samples and 16S ribosomal RNA (rRNA) genes are amplified using universal bacterial primers. This approach allows in theory amplification of DNA from all known and unknown bacterial species present in a sample. To identify the phylotypes present in the sample, the PCR amplicons can be subsequently sequenced by high-throughput sequencing platforms.[6] These platforms allow for analysis of several thousand sequences within a few hours, yielding a deep identification of the intestinal microbiota. If the sequence for a particular phylotype is known, specific PCR assays can be designed for its detection. Real-time polymerase chain reaction (PCR) assays (with universal-specific, group-specific, or species-specific primers) can be used for quantitative analysis. Fluorescent in situ hybridization (FISH) allows visualization of the location of bacteria with regard to the epithelium (ie, intracellular, adherent, or invasive).[7]

INTESTINAL MICROBIOTA OF MAMMALS
Humans, Mice, Dogs, Cats

Most data are available about the microbiota of humans and their animal models and, in veterinary medicine, about dogs and cats. These data are briefly summarized here as a reference for comparison with exotic and avian species. There is a remarkable similarity in the predominant bacterial phyla present in the GI tract across carnivores and omnivores, and also along the length of the GI tract.[8] The predominant phyla in the feces of healthy dogs, cats, and humans are Bacteroidetes, Firmicutes, Fusobacteria, and Proteobacteria.[1,8,9] On lower phylogenetic levels, the small intestine of dogs harbors predominantly Clostridia, Lactobacillales, and various classes of Proteobacteria, whereas the large intestine harbors almost exclusively anaerobic species from the orders of Clostridiales and Bacteroides, the families Ruminococcaceae and Lachnospiraceae, and the genera *Prevotella* and *Fusobacteria*.[8] Members of the Clostridiales order are especially highly abundant and it is thought that the bacterial species within this order perform major functions in the large intestine, such as the production of SCFA, indole metabolism, vitamin synthesis, and amino acid synthesis.[10] Although the intestine also harbors various resident fungi[6,11] and viruses,[1] little is currently known about their contribution to health and disease.

Rabbits, Ferrets, and Hamsters

Fewer studies have been reported characterizing the intestinal microbiota of other animal species, and even less is known about the metabolic functions of these gut communities compared with the previously described animal species. Studies characterizing the microbiota of rabbits have described mostly bacteria in fecal or cecal samples, and only limited information is available about the bacterial composition in the stomach and small intestine. Some of these studies observed many yet uncharacterized bacterial sequences in the rabbit's large intestine, suggesting that rabbits have a more unique microbial ecosystem compared with other animal species. Given the emerging importance of the gut microbiota for host health, there is need for more comprehensive descriptive studies cataloging the intestinal microbiota and their functional capacity in exotic animals. Rabbits are hindgut fermenters and seem to have microbiota similar to horses because both harbor large proportions of *Streptococcus* and Verrucomicrobia in fecal samples.[12,13] Published studies describing the known bacterial taxa reported the predominance of Clostridia (especially Ruminococcaceae and Lachnospiraceae), Bacteroidetes, and *Akkermansia* in rabbits.[14–17]

In a recent study, the fecal microbiota of ferrets was analyzed using the bacterial cultivation method. The predominant bacterial groups were *Clostridium acetobutylicum*, *Helicobacter* spp, and *Lactobacillus* spp.[18] To the author's knowledge, no molecular-based study was reported in literature describing the intestinal microbiota of ferrets. Therefore, it is likely that the intestinal microbiota of ferrets harbors many others besides the reported bacterial taxa. One study described the cecal microbiota of hamsters and found that Firmicutes, especially Clostridiales (families Ruminococcaceae and Lachnospiraceae) were most abundant.[19] Of interest is that fasting, but not hibernation, led to significant changes in gut microbiota, especially increases in the abundance of mucin-degrading bacteria such as *Akkermansia muciniphila*.[19] It has also been recently shown in dogs that prolonged fasting has a very strong impact on the small intestinal microbiota.[20] These initial studies describing the intestinal microbiota of small mammals suggest that the microbiota is as complex as in larger mammals, warranting more in-depth studies evaluating the intestinal microbiota across various diseases, and before and after nutritional interventions.

INTESTINAL MICROBIOTA OF PARROTS AND PSITTACINES

Compared with the many studies that have been performed in humans and other mammalian species, little information is yet available about the intestinal microbiota of birds beyond chickens. Similarly, very little information is available about the differences in microbiota composition along the intestinal tract and luminal versus mucosal-adherent bacterial populations. In one of the first molecular-based studies, the cloacal microbiota of 16 parrots (mealy Amazon parrot and macaws) was analyzed: 8 parrots were free-ranging in southeastern Peru and 8 parrots were living in captivity in a colony in Texas.[21] In this initial small-scale study, there was a trend for clustering of the captive birds versus the wild birds and, in the captive birds, based on the species and/or aviary they came from. Four predominant phyla were present across these cloacal samples in descending order of abundance: Firmicutes, Proteobacteria, Actinobacteria, and Bacteroidetes. On lower phylogenetic levels, the bacterial families Lactobacillaceae and Staphylococcaceae were predominant. In a recently reported large-scale study, the fecal microbiota of 3 different avian species (budgerigars, cockatiels, and domestic canaries) was analyzed by next-generation sequencing of 16S rRNA genes.[22] Firmicutes were the most abundant bacterial phylum, followed by Proteobacteria and Actinobacteria. *Lactobacillus* spp was the most abundant genus across all birds. Of interest was that the microbiota composition tended to be more similar for each bird species, suggesting that birds within an avian species have more similar microbiota compared with birds of other avian species.[22] Similarly, a recent study described the fecal microbiota of captive cockatiels, and reported that Firmicutes were most abundant, comprising mostly Erysipelotrichaceae, *Clostridium* and *Lactobacillus* spp, respectively.[23] These studies suggest that avian species have, in part, a different microbiota compared with mammals because they appear to have relative higher abundances of *Lactobacillus* spp.

To better understand the microbiota composition and its contribution for immune regulation, nutrition, and metabolism of birds, more descriptive studies are clearly needed about the intestinal microbiota (especially across the various avian species) and about the microbiota along the intestinal tract. In a study (Rossi and colleagues, unpublished data, 2014) from the author's laboratory, initial data suggest that crop and cloaca harbor similar species richness but very distinct microbial communities (ie, different makeup of bacterial taxa). Proteobacteria were significantly more abundant in the crop compared with the cloaca, whereas Firmicutes (mostly *Lactobacillus* spp) and Actinobacteria were more abundant in the cloaca. This distribution is similar, at least in part, to that described in mammals, in which aerobic bacteria, such as Proteobacteria, are more abundant in more proximal parts of the GI tract, and Firmicutes are more abundant more distally.[8] The reader is referred to other review articles that provide an overview about microbiota composition across other bird species.[24–26]

EXAMPLES OF GUT-BRAIN AXIS INTERACTIONS ACROSS ANIMAL MODELS

Until recently, the main focus for examining intestinal bacteria was to search for potential enteropathogens associated with various intestinal diseases. Just as with the appreciation of the close relationship between intestinal microbiota and the host, the investigators realized that gut microbiota composition also influences organ systems beyond the GI tract, and is associated with changes in cognition, behavior, stress, and other disorders of the nervous system.[27,28] One potential pathway is the direct immunologic stimulation through cell-to-cell contact affecting the enteric nervous or immune system that then further provides stimulatory signals to the brain. Another potential pathway is the production of endocrine metabolites by the intestinal microbiota that, in turn, stimulate the nervous system. Although those stimuli are physiologic and beneficial, negative effects can occur when there are imbalances in commensal microbiota because they may occur through external triggers (eg, use of antibiotics), through nutritional imbalances, and also through intestinal inflammation, which, in turn, affects microbiota composition. Examples from the literature across different animal models are summarized here to provide a broad overview about the current knowledge in the field.

Specific members of the microbiota have been shown to directly produce neurotransmitters, such as gamma-aminobutyric acid (GABA) or acetylcholine, under in vitro conditions. It is likely that this may also occur within the GI tract.[29] It was reported that there is a significant difference in the production of neuroendocrine substances (eg, catecholamines, norepinephrine, and dopamine) between mice that are born under normal conditions with a commensal microbiota versus mice that were born and remained germfree (ie, mice that were never exposed to intestinal microbes). These neuroendocrine substances were detected in the normal mice at regular concentrations but at much lower concentrations in the germfree mice, suggesting that the intestinal microbiota produces significant amounts of these neuroendocrine substances.[30] On the other side, neuroendocrine substances produced by the host during periods of stress may modulate the virulence of enteropathogens in vivo, providing evidence how host neuroendocrine substances have also an effect on gut microbiota.[31]

There is also clear evidence that GI colonization with potential enteropathogens can alter the behavior of the infected animals.[32] For example, in 1 study, mice were inoculated with *Campylobacter jejuni*, leading to mild subclinical infection that did not lead to measurable activation of the immune system (ie, no alterations in proinflammatory cytokine expression).[32] Nevertheless, the infected mice showed increases in anxiety, which manifested itself through a decrease in exploratory behavior, suggesting that the microbiota directly activated neural pathways.[32] Subsequent follow-up work by the same investigators revealed that the colonization with *C jejuni* indeed activated the nucleus of the solitary tract and the lateral parabrachial nucleus in the brainstem, supporting evidence that the gut reacts to the subclinical infection and then further signals to the brain.[33]

Some neurologic disorders have been associated with changes in the global commensal microbiota composition, rather than an infection with an external pathogen. For example, multiple sclerosis in humans has repeatedly been linked to altered microbial communities in the gut,[34] especially increases in *Methanobrevibacter* and *Akkermansia* and decreases in *Prevotella*.[35] Similarly, a recent study analyzed the fecal microbiota of dogs with meningoencephalomyelitis of unknown origin (MUO), which is an immune-mediated condition of dogs that has been suggested as a potential model for studying the pathophysiology of multiple sclerosis in humans.[36] Fecal samples were obtained from 20 dogs that were diagnosed with MUO and the microbiota was compared with the 20 control dogs accurately matched for breed, age, and gender. As observed in humans with multiple sclerosis, Prevotellaceae were significantly less abundant in dogs with MUO, providing additional evidence that presence of Prevotellaceae at higher abundances are associated with reduced risk for developing immune-mediated brain disease.[36]

Autism spectrum disorders (ASDs) are other neurodevelopmental diseases with emerging evidence for the role of the gut microbiota.[37] Human patients with ASD exhibit neurologic and, often, GI disorders. Several studies have reported alterations in gut microbiota in people with ASD compared with controls.[37,38] Furthermore, therapeutic manipulation of the gut microbiota in children with ASD revealed improvements in GI and behavioral symptoms of ASD.[39] In a small open-label pilot study, 18 children diagnosed with ASD received an initial 2-week treatment with a nonabsorbable antibiotic, followed by a bowel cleanse. These children then received fecal microbiota transplantation daily for 7 to 8 weeks.[39] The symptoms of children improved during therapy with lasting effect even after completion of therapy, suggesting a prolonged change in gut microbiota associated with improvement of ASD.

Bacterial components have also been shown to directly modulate brain development and, subsequently, behavior. For example, in 1 study, bacterial peptidoglycan (PGN) was derived from the commensal gut microbiota and it was shown that PGN was able to translocate into the brain and was sensed by specific pattern-recognition receptors within the innate immune system.[40] Furthermore, the absence of these bacterial factors was associated with increased risk for autism-like behavior in a mouse model. Similarly, in mice, polysaccharide A from the capsule of the commensal bacterium *Bacteroides fragilis* was protective of experimental autoimmune encephalomyelitis, which is the experimental model of human multiple sclerosis.[41] The proposed mechanism was due to induction of immunoregulatory T cells by the polysaccharide A capsule. Of importance is that this protective effect was not induced by all strains of *B fragilis* but only by the specific strain *B fragilis* (ATCC 9343).[42] The effect is believed to be due to enhancement of gut barrier function.

Nutrition also plays a role by modulating gut microbiota, which, in turn, affects cognition and behavior. For example, feeding of resistant starch to mice revealed that animals developed more pronounced anxiety-like behavior.[43] Mood disorders have been associated with dietary sensitivities that were hypothesized to be caused by increased gut permeability due to infectious agents such as *Toxoplasma gondii*, influenzavirus, and coronavirus.[44] Nutrition and carbohydrate catabolism due to microbial metabolism in the small intestine was also associated with autism syndrome disorders in humans.[45] There are a variety of changes at the genus and species level found in the duodenal microbiota in children with autism that could potentially be caused by carbohydrate malabsorption. These observations may represent a pronounced and enduring dysbiosis that results in formation of metabolites that affect the behavior of autistic children.[45]

SUMMARY

Studies have shown strong evidence for a bidirectional link between gut microbiota and the brain. So far, most studies have shown mechanistic links in mouse models of disease. However, the first therapeutic pilot trials in children with autism provide support for the notion that manipulation of gut microbiota may be an important pathway for future therapies. This is an exciting area of research and highlights the need for more comprehensive studies to better define the intestinal microbiota in mammals and avian species. Future therapeutic trials will be necessary to evaluate how diet, probiotics, and even fecal microbiota transplantation may be used for establishing an optimal microbiota. Also, recent studies have shown the detrimental long-term impact of antibiotics on the gut microbiota, which should alert clinicians to use antibiotics more judiciously.

REFERENCES

1. Swanson KS, Dowd SE, Suchodolski JS, et al. Phylogenetic and gene-centric metagenomics of the canine intestinal microbiome reveals similarities with humans and mice. ISME J 2011;5(4):639–49.
2. Rondeau MP, Meltzer K, Michel KE, et al. Short chain fatty acids stimulate feline colonic smooth muscle contraction. J Feline Med Surg 2003;5(3):167–73.
3. Scheppach W. Effects of short chain fatty acids on gut morphology and function. Gut 1994;35(Suppl. 1):S35–8.
4. Arpaia N, Campbell C, Fan X, et al. Metabolites produced by commensal bacteria promote peripheral regulatory T-cell generation. Nature 2013;504(7480): 451–5.
5. Bansal T, Alaniz RC, Wood TK, et al. The bacterial signal indole increases epithelial-cell tight-junction resistance and attenuates indicators of inflammation. Proc Natl Acad Sci U S A 2010;107(1):228–33.
6. Handl S, Dowd SE, Garcia-Mazcorro JF, et al. Massive parallel 16S rRNA gene pyrosequencing reveals highly diverse fecal bacterial and fungal communities in healthy dogs and cats. FEMS Microbiol Ecol 2011;76(2):301–10.
7. Simpson KW, Dogan B, Rishniw M, et al. Adherent and invasive Escherichia coli is associated with granulomatous colitis in boxer dogs. Infect Immun 2006;74(8): 4778–92.
8. Honneffer JB. Variation of the microbiota and metabolome along the canine gastrointestinal tract. Metabolomics 2017;13:26.
9. Suchodolski JS, Foster ML, Sohail MU, et al. The fecal microbiome in cats with diarrhea. PLoS One 2015;10(5):e0127378.
10. Guard BC, Suchodolski JS. Horse Species Symposium: canine intestinal microbiology and metagenomics: From phylogeny to function. J Anim Sci 2016;94(6): 2247–61.
11. Suchodolski JS, Morris EK, Allenspach K, et al. Prevalence and identification of fungal DNA in the small intestine of healthy dogs and dogs with chronic enteropathies. Vet Microbiol 2008;132(3–4):379–88.
12. Steelman SM, Chowdhary BP, Dowd S, et al. Pyrosequencing of 16S rRNA genes in fecal samples reveals high diversity of hindgut microflora in horses and potential links to chronic laminitis. BMC Vet Res 2012;8:231.
13. Costa MC, Arroyo LG, Allen-Vercoe E, et al. Comparison of the fecal microbiota of healthy horses and horses with colitis by high throughput sequencing of the V3-V5 region of the 16S rRNA gene. PLoS One 2012;7(7):e41484.
14. Zeng B, Han S, Wang P, et al. The bacterial communities associated with fecal types and body weight of rex rabbits. Scientific Rep 2015;5:9342.
15. Eshar D, Weese JS. Molecular analysis of the microbiota in hard feces from healthy rabbits (Oryctolagus cuniculus) medicated with long term oral meloxicam. BMC Vet Res 2014;10:62.
16. Bauerl C, Collado MC, Zuniga M, et al. Changes in cecal microbiota and mucosal gene expression revealed new aspects of epizootic rabbit enteropathy. PLoS One 2014;9(8):e105707.
17. Combes S, Michelland RJ, Monteils V, et al. Postnatal development of the rabbit caecal microbiota composition and activity. FEMS Microbiol Ecol 2011;77(3): 680–9.
18. Nizza S, Rando F, Fiorito F, et al. Fecal microbiota and antibiotic resistance in ferrets (Mustela putorius furo) from two captive breeding facilities in Italy. Res Vet Sci 2014;96(3):426–8.

19. Sonoyama K, Fujiwara R, Takemura N, et al. Response of gut microbiota to fasting and hibernation in Syrian hamsters. Appl Environ Microbiol 2009;75(20):6451–6.
20. Kasiraj AC, Harmoinen J, Isaiah A, et al. The effects of feeding and withholding food on the canine small intestinal microbiota. FEMS Microbiol Ecol 2016;92(6): fiw085.
21. Xenoulis PG, Gray PL, Brightsmith D, et al. Molecular characterization of the cloacal microbiota of wild and captive parrots. Vet Microbiol 2010;146(3–4): 320–5.
22. Garcia-Mazcorro JF, Castillo-Carranza SA, Guard B, et al. Comprehensive molecular characterization of bacterial communities in feces of pet birds using 16S Marker Sequencing. Microb Ecol 2017;73(1):224–35.
23. Alcaraz LD, Hernandez AM, Peimbert M. Exploring the cockatiel (*Nymphicus hollandicus*) fecal microbiome, bacterial inhabitants of a worldwide pet. PeerJ 2016; 4:e2837.
24. Kohl KD. Diversity and function of the avian gut microbiota. J Comp Physiol B 2012;182(5):591–602.
25. Waite DW, Taylor MW. Exploring the avian gut microbiota: current trends and future directions. Front Microbiol 2015;6:673.
26. Waite DW, Taylor MW. Characterizing the avian gut microbiota: membership, driving influences, and potential function. Front Microbiol 2014;5:223.
27. Montiel-Castro AJ, Gonzalez-Cervantes RM, Bravo-Ruiseco G, et al. The microbiota-gut-brain axis: neurobehavioral correlates, health and sociality. Front Integr Neurosci 2013;7:70.
28. Martin CR, Mayer EA. Gut-brain axis and behavior. Nestle Nutr Inst Workshop Ser 2017;88:45–53.
29. Barrett E, Ross RP, O'Toole PW, et al. γ-Aminobutyric acid production by culturable bacteria from the human intestine. J Appl Microbiol 2012;113(2):411–7.
30. Asano Y, Hiramoto T, Nishino R, et al. Critical role of gut microbiota in the production of biologically active, free catecholamines in the gut lumen of mice. Am J Physiol Gastrointest Liver Physiol 2012;303(11):G1288–95.
31. Pullinger GD, Carnell SC, Sharaff FF, et al. Norepinephrine augments *Salmonella enterica*-induced enteritis in a manner associated with increased net replication but independent of the putative adrenergic sensor kinases QseC and QseE. Infect Immun 2010;78(1):372–80.
32. Lyte M, Varcoe JJ, Bailey MT. Anxiogenic effect of subclinical bacterial infection in mice in the absence of overt immune activation. Physiol Behav 1998;65(1):63–8.
33. Gaykema RP, Goehler LE, Lyte M. Brain response to cecal infection with *Campylobacter jejuni*: analysis with Fos immunohistochemistry. Brain Behav Immun 2004;18(3):238–45.
34. Jangi S, Gandhi R, Cox LM, et al. Alterations of the human gut microbiome in multiple sclerosis. Nat Commun 2016;7:12015.
35. Chen J, Chia N, Kalari KR, et al. Multiple sclerosis patients have a distinct gut microbiota compared to healthy controls. Scientific Rep 2016;6:28484.
36. Jeffery ND, Barker AK, Alcott CJ, et al. The association of specific constituents of the fecal microbiota with immune-mediated brain disease in dogs. PLoS One 2017;12(1):e0170589.
37. Strati F, Cavalieri D, Albanese D, et al. New evidences on the altered gut microbiota in autism spectrum disorders. Microbiome 2017;5(1):24.
38. Berding K, Donovan SM. Microbiome and nutrition in autism spectrum disorder: current knowledge and research needs. Nutr Rev 2016;74(12):723–36.

39. Kang DW, Adams JB, Gregory AC, et al. Microbiota Transfer Therapy alters gut ecosystem and improves gastrointestinal and autism symptoms: an open-label study. Microbiome 2017;5(1):10.
40. Arentsen T, Qian Y, Gkotzis S, et al. The bacterial peptidoglycan-sensing molecule Pglyrp2 modulates brain development and behavior. Mol Psychiatry 2017; 22(2):257–66.
41. Ochoa-Reparaz J, Mielcarz DW, Ditrio LE, et al. Central nervous system demyelinating disease protection by the human commensal *Bacteroides fragilis* depends on polysaccharide A expression. J Immunol 2010;185(7):4101–8.
42. Ochoa-Reparaz J, Mielcarz DW, Wang Y, et al. A polysaccharide from the human commensal *Bacteroides fragilis* protects against CNS demyelinating disease. Mucosal Immunol 2010;3(5):487–95.
43. Lyte M, Chapel A, Lyte JM, et al. Resistant starch alters the microbiota-gut brain axis: implications for dietary modulation of behavior. PLoS One 2016;11(1): e0146406.
44. Casella G, Pozzi R, Cigognetti M, et al. Mood disorders and non-celiac gluten sensitivity. Minerva Gastroenterol Dietol 2017;63(1):32–7.
45. Kushak RI, Winter HS, Buie TM, et al. Analysis of the duodenal microbiome in autistic individuals: association with carbohydrate digestion. J Pediatr Gastroenterol Nutr 2017;64(5):e110–6.

Moving?

Make sure your subscription moves with you!

To notify us of your new address, find your **Clinics Account Number** (located on your mailing label above your name), and contact customer service at:

Email: journalscustomerservice-usa@elsevier.com

800-654-2452 (subscribers in the U.S. & Canada)
314-447-8871 (subscribers outside of the U.S. & Canada)

Fax number: 314-447-8029

**Elsevier Health Sciences Division
Subscription Customer Service
3251 Riverport Lane
Maryland Heights, MO 63043**

*To ensure uninterrupted delivery of your subscription, please notify us at least 4 weeks in advance of move.

Moving?

Make sure your subscription moves with you!

To notify us of your new address, find your Clinics Account Number (located on your mailing label above your name), and contact customer service at:

Email: journalscustomerservice-usa@elsevier.com

800-654-2452 (subscribers in the U.S. & Canada)
314-447-8871 (subscribers outside of the U.S. & Canada)

Fax number: 314-447-8029

Elsevier Health Sciences Division
Subscription Customer Service
3251 Riverport Lane
Maryland Heights, MO 63043